The BMA Family Doctor Guides

Strokes and their Prevention

Titles in the series:

Confusion in Old Age
Gallstones and Liver Problems
Arthritis
Asthma
Children's Health 1–5
Strokes and their Prevention

John Morris

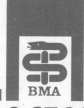

FAMILY DOCTOR GUIDES

Strokes and their Prevention

Dr D.J. Thomas

Series editor: Dr Tony Smith

Dr Thomas is consultant neurologist at St Mary's Hospital, Paddington, and the National Hospital for Nervous Diseases, London

Published by Equation in association with the British Medical Association.

First published 1988

© British Medical Association 1988

All rights reserved. No part of this publication may be
reproduced, stored in a retrieval system, or transmitted
in any form or by any means, electronic, mechanical,
photocopying, or otherwise, without prior permission in
writing from the publishers.

British Library Cataloguing in Publication Data

Thomas, J. D.
Strokes and their prevention.
1. Man. Brain. Strokes
I. Title   II. Series
616.8'1

ISBN 1-85336-078-3

Picture acknowledgements
John Rae: pp. 12, 27, 37, 44, 53, 67, 70, 88; Dept. Medical
Illustrations, St. Bartholomew's Hospital: pp. 21, 22, 50; Westminster
Hospital CT Scanning Unit: p. 46; Family Planning Association:
p. 95; David Woodroffe: diagrams; Derek Marriott: cartoons.

Equation, Wellingborough, Northamptonshire NN8 2RQ, England

Typeset by Columns of Reading
Printed and bound in Great Britain by The Bath Press, Avon

10 9 8 7 6 5 4 3 2 1

Contents

1 INTRODUCTION   7
   What are the causes?; An important medical
   problem; The aims of the book

2 SOME BASIC ANATOMY   9
   What determines the degree of disability; What
   do cerebral hemispheres do?; What does the
   brain stem do?; The cerebellum; The spinal
   cord; Blood supply (circulation)

3 WHAT GOES WRONG?   17
   What causes a cerebral infarct?; More about
   cerebral thrombosis; Cerebral embolism;
   Intracranial haemorrhage; Importance of site
   and size; Cerebral swelling (oedema);
   Causes of death; A better outlook for some

4 CLINICAL FEATURES OF A STROKE   26
   One week later...; What caused the stroke?;
   Consciousness level; Weakness; Speech;
   Damaged thought processes; Sensory
   disturbances; Sight; Other possible problems;
   Continence

5 COMMON COMPLICATIONS AFTER A STROKE   39
   Frozen shoulder; Deep vein thrombosis and
   pulmonary emboli; Pneumonia; Bed sores;
   Convulsions; Emotional problems

6 TESTS AND INVESTIGATIONS   45
   The brain; The blood; Investigation of the arteries;
   Non-invasive investigations; Angiography; The heart

7 TREATMENT WHEN A STROKE OCCURS   52
   Breathing and swallowing; Convulsions; Heart
   problems; Deep vein thrombosis; Antiplatelet
   and anticoagulant therapy; Changes in the
   blood; Blood pressure problems; Treating
   complications; Surgical treatment; Nursing
   care and other specialist therapies;
   Morale; Treatment of the future

8 AFTER THE FIRST TWO WEEKS   64
Prospects; Order of recovery; After six months;
Up to two years; Nursing care; Physiotherapy;
Speech therapy; Occupational therapy;
Medical social worker; Rehabilitation units;
Most patients go home

9 GOING HOME   74
But support is needed; Improving facilities
at home; The GP takes over; Diet; Medication;
Emotional problems; Intellectual difficulties;
Resuming contact with others; Returning to
work; Back into the driving seat; Sex after
stroke; Conclusion

10 CARERS NEED CARE TOO   84
Let others help; Don't bottle up your feelings;
Holidays should help; If you can't cope

11 RISK FACTORS FOR STROKE   86
Factors apply to other problems; Previous signs;
Age; High blood pressure; Transient cerebral
ischaemic attacks; Heart disease; High
cholesterol; Diabetes mellitus; Thickness of
the blood; Overweight; Smoking; Alcohol;
The oral contraceptive pill; The role of stress;
Family history; A thorough check-up?

12 PREVENTING STROKE   98
Secondary prevention; Primary prevention; The
patient with no risk factors

USEFUL NAMES AND ADDRESSES   104

GLOSSARY   106

INDEX   109

1 Introduction

A stroke is something we all dread, but most of us are not quite sure what it is. Although we probably know that a stroke means a sudden paralysis of one side of the body and possibly speech disturbance, there is often more to it, as this book will explain.

What are the causes?

The most common cause is a cerebral thrombosis. A blood clot (thrombus) blocks one of the blood vessels supplying the brain causing damage to that part of the brain. The other causes of stroke include bleeding into the brain (cerebral haemorrhage) and blocking of blood vessels in the brain by clots from other parts of the circulatory system (cerebral embolism). Occasionally patients with brain tumours may have the same sort of symptoms are those who have had a stroke (see p. 20).

An important medical problem

Stroke is a very major medical problem in this country and it is second only to heart attacks as a cause of death. About one in three of us will have a stroke and one in seven of us may die from it.

A stroke may be a disaster for both the sufferer and his family. It may be impossible to return to work afterwards: it may even be impossible to communicate with others or to look after oneself. Stroke is the commonest cause of disability in middle aged and elderly people, and providing long term care for the more severely disabled is a tremendous challenge for both families and society. Another distressing fact is that those who have had several strokes are more likely to develop a dementing illness in which there is a progressive decline in their mental abilities.

The aims of this book

This book will try:
- To help you understand more about strokes;
- To enable you to cope more easily if you or a relative or friend have a stroke;
- To teach you how to prevent a stroke in the first place, or a recurrence if you have already had one.

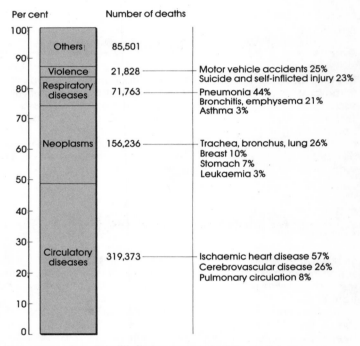

Major cause of death in UK. Stroke accounts for 25% of all deaths.

Glossary

There is a list of medical terms and their meanings at the end of the book.

2 Some basic anatomy

Some simple anatomy will help you to understand a stroke better, but you may skip this section if you find it too complicated and move straight on to p. 17. For our present purposes, the brain can be considered as being made up of the two cerebral hemispheres, the brain stem, and the cerebellum. The brain stem is the thin structure which continues down the back as the spinal cord. The messages to and from the limbs and the body and the cerebral hemispheres are conducted via the spinal cord and the brain stem. There is free communication between the cerebellum, which is concerned with coordination, and the brain stem and therefore with the cerebral hemispheres and the spinal cord and arms and legs.

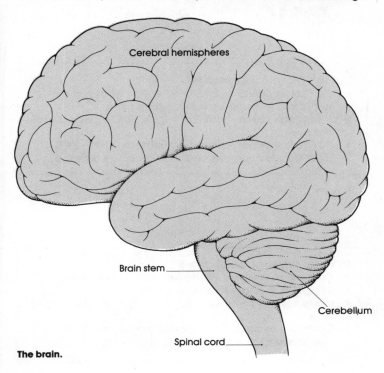

The brain.

What determines the degree of disability

The amount of disability caused by a stroke depends on the site at which it strikes, how much damage there is, and also on how the complicated interactions between the damaged area and the other parts of the brain are affected. Damage to these interactions may cause more complex problems than simple paralysis or loss of sensation. For example, patients recovering from a stroke may find their main problem is that they are not able to use their limbs appropriately. They may have lost the skills they have learnt such as being able to wash, comb their hair, or dress themselves (called 'apraxia'); or they may be unable to recognise people or things (called 'agnosia').

What do the cerebral hemispheres do?

The left cerebral hemisphere
- **Controls movement of the right side of the body;**
- **Interprets feelings from the right side;**
- **Interprets vision from the right half of the visual field;**
- **Controls speech and understanding in 99% of right handed people and in 60% of left handers.**

The right cerebral hemisphere
- **Controls movement of the left side of the body;**
- **Interprets feelings from the left side;**
- **Interprets vision from the left side of the visual field;**
- **Controls speech in approximately 40% of left handers and in only 1% of right handers.**

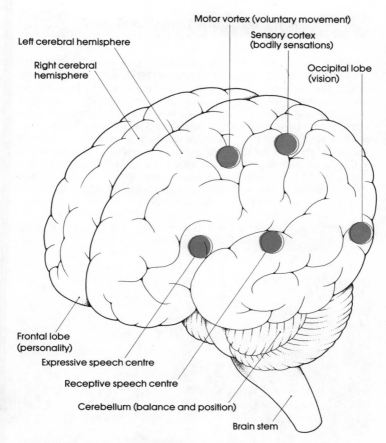

Left cerebral hemisphere

Right cerebral hemisphere

Motor vortex (voluntary movement)

Sensory cortex (bodily sensations)

Occipital lobe (vision)

Frontal lobe (personality)

Expressive speech centre

Receptive speech centre

Cerebellum (balance and position)

Brain stem

The left and right cerebral hemispheres of the brain.

Input and output

In general terms, the front half of each cerebral hemisphere is concerned with output – it governs movement, expressive speech, and planning, including simple tasks like washing and dressing. The rear half of the hemisphere is concerned with input, such as bodily sensations and vision and also with the interpretation of these. Clearly, coordinated action needs rapid communication within each hemisphere and between the two hemispheres (via the 'corpus callosum').

What does the brain stem do?

Because the brain stem passes messages to and from the brain, a stroke that strikes this part may also cause paralysis and disturbed sensations on one side of the body. In addition, however, the brain stem has functions of its own. In particular, it is concerned with eye movements and with consciousness – consider the everyday experience of the association of eyes and sleep. Furthermore, it is concerned with vital functions that we so often take for granted until a problem arises – functions such as swallowing, ability to clear the throat and coughing, and also with the formation of words and the quality of speech rather than its content. The speech of someone who has had a stroke may be so distorted because of difficulties with articulation, that although he knows exactly what he wants to say, no-one else can understand him (this is called severe 'dysarthria').

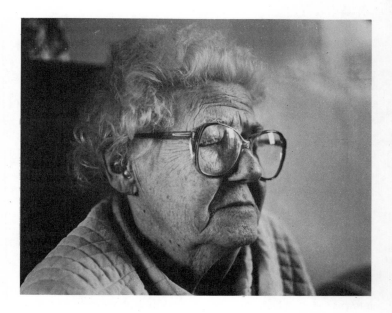

The brain stem is concerned with sleep.

The cerebellum

The cerebellum is concerned with coordination and balance and with the 'smoothing out' of movements that are commanded by the cerebral hemispheres. Damage to the cerebellum may therefore produce difficulty in walking, sometimes as if the patient were drunk, without there being any noticeable one-sided paralysis, or a tendency to fall backwards. Patients with problems in the cerebellum may often tremble so much whenever they reach for an object that they cannot grasp it.

The spinal cord

The spinal cord is only rarely the site of stroke. For some reason a blockage in one of the arteries supplying the spinal cord with blood occurs less commonly here than in other parts of the central nervous system. When there is a blockage, however, the patient usually suffers a sudden paralysis of both legs – a 'paraplegia.'

Blood supply (circulation)

The brain is extremely greedy for blood. It has a supply approximately ten times greater than that to our muscles and approximately a quarter of the blood pumped out by the heart goes to the brain.

The heart

The working of the heart has a very important influence on the circulation of blood to the brain. If your heart stops supplying enough blood to your brain, you will lose consciousness within seconds, and unless the blood supply is returned promptly, permanent brain damage or brain death will occur within just a few minutes. Faulty heart valves or a recent heart attack may result in blood clots forming in the heart. If those are dislodged and find their way to the brain they may cause a stroke.

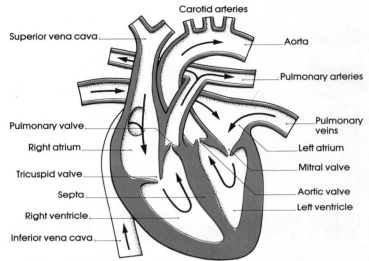

The heart showing position of carotid arteries.

Carotid and vertebral arteries

The blood supply to the brain is provided by two carotid arteries and two vertebral arteries. The carotid arteries carry approximately 70% of the total brain blood and the vertebral arteries the remaining 30%. The carotid arteries branch into the anterior and middle cerebral arteries, which supply the front of the cerebral hemispheres, except the visual cortex at the back of the head and the under-surfaces of both temporal lobes. These are supplied by the posterior cerebral arteries coming from the vertebral arteries.

The major blood vessels in the neck are very important because they are a common site for the development of narrowing of the arteries as a result of a disorder called arteriosclerosis ('hardening of the arteries'). The carotid arteries branch in the neck to form the internal carotid artery which supplies the brain and the external carotid artery which supplies the face and the neck. The beginning of the internal carotid artery is a particularly common site for narrowing to occur. The narrowing affects the blood flow and may cause a clot to develop. If this dislodges and shoots up the internal carotid artery to block one of the smaller arteries in the brain a stroke may occur. Fortunately arteriosclerosis of the carotid arteries can be treated surgically, with some success.

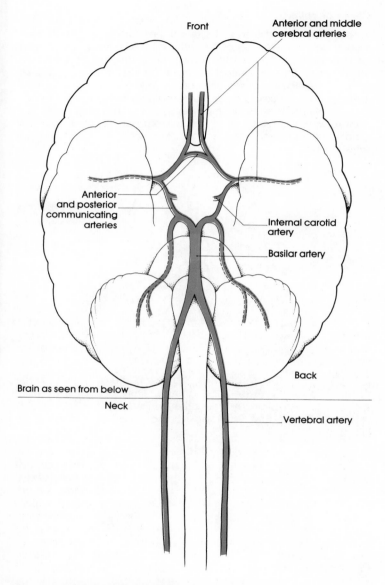

Front

Anterior and middle cerebral arteries

Anterior and posterior communicating arteries

Internal carotid artery

Basilar artery

Back

Brain as seen from below

Neck

Vertebral artery

The cerebral blood supply and arteries in the neck.

Circle of Willis

Inside the head, the four major arteries join in a roundabout system called the Circle of Willis. This allows blood to be shared around within the head to compensate for any neck movements, when flow up one of the neck arteries may fail. It is also useful if disease causes the blockage of one of the four feeding vessels. Blood from the remaining three neck arteries may continue to supply the whole of the brain through this communicating circle. It is not uncommon for one internal carotid or vertebral artery to be blocked without the patient suffering a stroke.

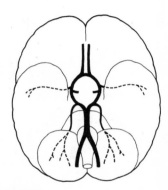

The Circle of Willis.

Beyond the Circle of Willis, however, there is very poor communication between the arteries. One part of the brain tends to be supplied by one artery and when this is blocked and the blood flow is stopped, that part of the brain is damaged.

3 What goes wrong?

Patients who seem to have suffered a stroke are likely to have had either blockage of a cerebral artery which causes death of an area of brain tissue (a cerebral infarct) or bleeding into the brain (an intracranial haemorrhage). Very occasionally, however, patients with a brain tumour may have a sudden paralysis, perhaps because they have bled from the tumour, have had a fit triggered by the tumour, or fluid has suddenly collected in the zone immediately around the tumour.

Cerebral infarct

In an infarct there is direct damage and death of brain tissue caused by a defect in the blood supply. In the centre of the damaged area, most of the brain cells may be dead but those nearer the edges, where blood from nearby arteries can reach, may survive.

Haemorrhage

In a brain haemorrhage, damage is slightly more complicated. Firstly, there is direct destruction of brain cells as a result of a sudden burst of blood into the delicate tissue. Secondly, the haemorrhage itself may then start to expand, which damages more brain cells by pressure, distortion, and displacement. Thirdly, the vessel that has bled often becomes blocked or narrowed by a blood clot and this will interefere with the blood supply to other areas of the brain.

What causes a cerebral infarct?

A cerebral infarct may be caused by:

- A thrombosis (blood clot) forming in a blood vessel in the brain (cerebral thrombosis);
- A cerebral embolism; where a blood clot forms elsewhere (for example, in the heart or in one of the major arteries supplying the brain), becomes dislodged, forms an embolus, moves up into the brain, and then becomes jammed in one of the cerebral arteries.

More about cerebral thrombosis

Cerebral thrombosis may be the result of a moderate or severe degree of arteriosclerosis (narrowing) of the cerebral arteries. This disorder is strongly linked with age, but it is also caused by high blood pressure and is associated with other risk factors like diabetes and high concentrations of fats, including cholesterol, in the blood stream.

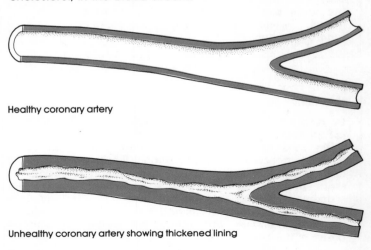

Healthy coronary artery

Unhealthy coronary artery showing thickened lining

Arteriosclerosis.

Diseased arteries

If you have diseased arteries, changes may occur in the way the blood flows and in the nature of the blood, and thrombosis may occur. We expect a lot of our blood. For over 100 years, in some cases, it is supposed to remain fluid in the circulation. Yet, within just five minutes of injury, a blood clot is expected to form to prevent further blood loss, and this clot needs to form just at the site of injury and not elsewhere in the body. It is not surprising therefore that the body gets it wrong at times, and when the inner surface of the artery is irregular or rough errors are more likely to occur.

How clots form

The platelets in the blood (thrombocytes) may get busy and stick to a roughened area on the inside of an artery. More thrombocytes may then become attached and changes in the blood fluid, plasma, take place which mean that eventually a thrombus (clot) is formed (this is known as the 'coagulation cascade'). Medical treatments to prevent such a disaster are aimed at reducing the stickiness and the activitiy of the platelets (antiplatelet therapy) or reducing the blood's ability to clot (anticoagulant treatment).

A thrombosis is much more likely to occur when the platelets have been stimulated and when the plasma is abnormal, for example as a result of injury or infection. Injury does include surgical treatment, and occasionally old people have a stroke after an operation. Patients sometimes suffer a stroke shortly after some other illness has increased the likelihood of thrombosis and there is some evidence that serious emotional stress can also increase the clotting tendency of the blood.

Cerebral embolism

An embolus is a clot of blood which is carried in the blood from another part of the body to the brain. The two most common sources for cerebral emboli are the heart and the carotid arteries. People who have had rheumatic fever and have diseased heart valves are vulnerable, particularly if they also have a disturbed heart rhythm (arrhythmia). Somewhat surprisingly, patients who have had a heart attack suffer relatively few strokes as a result of cerebral embolism. When they do, blood

19

clots formed over the damaged internal surface of the heart become dislodged and move to the aortic arch, the carotid arteries, and then to the head. These patients tend to do best on anticoagulant drug treatment rather than antiplatelet therapy.

Two case histories of real patients showing the problems that can arise. More case histories appear throughout the book.

Cerebellar Haemorrhage

A 60 year old peer of the realm suddenly became unsteady and unable to walk. He had severe headache and started vomiting. He was admitted to hospital with slurred speech and noticeable incoordination and his level of consciousness started to decline. He was found to have very high blood pressure and a haemorrhage in the cerebellum was suspected. An urgent brain scan was performed which confirmed the diagnosis. By this stage he was deeply unconscious and his breathing was becoming irregular. He was rushed to the operating theatre where a blood clot was removed. After the operation he had to be kept on a breathing machine for several days. Remobilisation was slow but after two months he was walking independently, albeit as if slightly drunk and not many months afterwards he was able to lead his daughter down the aisle at her wedding. He remains on drug treatment for his high blood pressure and the only remaining problems are minor slurring of his speech and momentary difficulty with balance when he turns quickly.

Brain tumour

A 48 year old housewife started to have frequent episodes in which, quite suddenly, she was unable to speak and she also had problems with understanding what was being said to her. She completely recovered within two to three minutes. The doctor thought she had been having transient cerebral ischaemic attacks and put her on aspirin. The attacks continued however, and dipyridamole was started but this made no difference. She was admitted to hospital urgently for investigation.

Examination showed subtle difficulties with speech and language function including minor problems with reading and writing even between her attacks. There were no abnormal noises over her heart or neck but a brain scan was performed which showed a tumour. This was found to be a benign tumour arising from the meninges (a meningioma) and was completely removed without any damage. The patient made a complete recovery and is not expected to have any further trouble of this nature.

Importance of the carotid arteries

The carotid arteries are of great practical importance not only because they are responsible for a stroke in a considerable number of patients, but also because they can be treated surgically. The most common site for narrowing of the carotid arteries is at the level of the jaw, where the common carotid artery divides into the internal carotid artery that supplies the brain and the external carotid artery supplying the face and neck. Patients with a problem at this site may have a short lived attack of weakness on one side of their body or speech disturbance lasting perhaps just a few minutes. This is called a transient ischaemic attack and may be the sign that a small thrombus has become dislodged from the diseased area. The concern is that a larger clot may form and become dislodged and that the patient will go on to have a more serious stroke rather than another transient ischaemic attack. The two current forms of treatment to prevent this happening are antiplatelet treatment to try to stop further platelet activity and the sticking of platelets to the diseased area and on operation called a carotid endarterectomy, which removes the partial blockage.

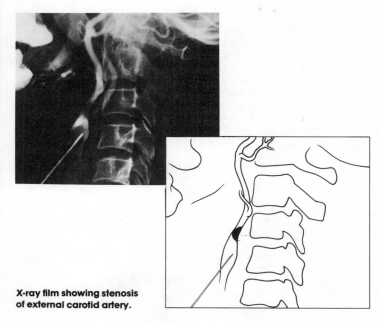

X-ray film showing stenosis of external carotid artery.

Intracranial haemorrhage

There are three major types of brain haemorrhage that can cause a stroke:

- Intracerebral haemorrhage (including bleeding into the cerebellum);
- Subarachnoid haemorrhage;
- Subdural haemorrhage.

Intracerebral haemorrhage

Intracerebral haemorrhage occurs when blood floods into the brain tissue itself from a burst blood vessel. The amount of bleeding may be small or large, depending on the size of the burst blood vessel and the efficiency with which the leak is sealed.

Subarachnoid haemorrhage

In subarachnoid haemorrhage, the site of the bleeding is different in that blood leaks between the membranes covering the brain – the meninges. It rapidly spreads over the surface of the brain rather than bursting into it. Subarachnoid haemorrhage causes very sudden, severe headache, sometimes with vomiting and loss of consciousness. When patients regain consciousness they have a stiff neck, dislike light, and, in milder cases, there is very little in the way of paralysis.

Patients who have suffered a subarachnoid haemorrhage

Berry aneurysm.

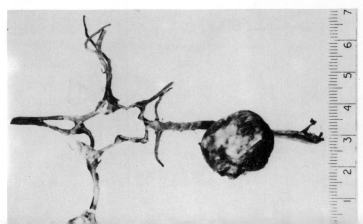

are often found to have a small swelling or sac (aneurysm) on one of the blood vessels in the brain, which has been caused by a weakening or stretching of that vessel. This is called a berry aneurysm and can often be treated surgically. Patients who have suffered a more severe haemorrhage and who have been weakened considerably are not good candidates for surgery and need more conservative treatment.

The blood that bathes the brain in a subarachnoid haemorrhage starts to break down after a few hours and the substances produced are irritative and may cause the blood vessels to go 'into spasm', which considerably increases the likelihood of further brain damage.

Subdural haemorrhage

This is caused by a head injury, lies immediately under the skull and is easily removed surgically.

Importance of site and size

The size and the location in the brain of a stroke determine how much functional loss the victim suffers. Small infarcts or haemorrhages in the cerebral hemispheres are not a threat to life and may not even affect function or independence if they are in relatively silent parts of the hemispheres, for example in the frontal or temporal lobes of the non-dominant hemisphere. Even small problems within the brainstem, however, may be very damaging. Here major nerve pathways and vital structures connected with swallowing and consciousness are packed closely together and the amount of functional loss is quite out of proportion to the size of the disturbance.

Size

Large infarcts or haemorrhages affecting the brain stem rapidly cause death. If these affect the cerebral hemispheres it is obvious that the patient has had a large stroke immediately after the event has occurred. Large strokes tend to cause a lot of brain swelling, which adds to the patient's disability and in some cases leads to their deterioration and death.

Cerebral swelling (oedema)

Cerebral swelling, or oedema, is caused by excess water which develops in the brain as a result of disease. The cerebral oedema that develops around a brain tumour responds very well to treatment with steroid drugs, at least in the short term, but these drugs do not have the same effect in stroke, which is a great disappointment.

In a brain tumour, the oedema develops as a result of water leaking from the blood vessels around the tumour. The normal division between the circulatory system and the brain tissue – the blood-brain barrier – is damaged and the extra water lies in the space between the blood vessels and the brain cells themselves. It is believed that steroid treatment restores the blood-brain barrier, prevents further leakage of fluid, and aids the reabsorption of fluid already there.

In stroke, the blood-brain barrier is also damaged and cerebral oedema occurs. The main problem however, is with the brain cells themselves – they become very swollen and do not improve with steroid therapy.

Increased pressure

The accumulation of excess water inside the closed box of the skull causes a rise in its internal pressure. This increased pressure threatens the blood supply in the immediate neighbourhood of the stroke and elsewhere inside the brain still further. In an attempt to achieve the same blood supply to the brain, the pressure in the unaffected arteries has to rise and this is one of the reasons why blood pressure increases after you have had a stroke.

A tight squeeze

The development of oedema leads to further squashing and movement of the brain tissues causing further disturbance of function. This is usually at its worst between the third and fifth day after a stroke and explains why many patients are at their lowest at this time.

Oedema is serious

Cerebral oedema is a major cause of death after a stroke. The affected cerebral hemisphere expands and part of it is pushed down through the hole in the tight membrane which separates the cerebellum from the cerebral hemisphere. Here it squeezes the brain stem. The patient starts to become drowsy, then unconscious, and may eventually stop breathing as a result of brain stem failure.

Causes of death

About a third of patients die soon after stroke and clearly, elderly patients have a higher chance of dying than younger and otherwise fit patients. The cause of death is often a massive stroke with associated cerebral oedema causing secondary pressure on the brain stem which results, as we have seen, in increasing unconsciousness and inability to breath. Sometimes, however, death occurs suddenly as a result of a large haemorrhage or infarct in the brain stem itself.

Deep vein thrombosis

Other causes of death include pulmonary emboli (blood clots in the lung) which may be the result of a deep vein thrombosis (clot in the vein) in the leg paralysed by the stroke. Deep vein thrombosis may occur in up to 40% of patients after a stroke, but only a small proportion of these will be unlucky enough to have a blood clot dislodge and move to the lung. Some people have a heart attack (myocardial infarct) in the early days after a stroke. As a result of being unable to move they may develop pneumonia and infections from the urinary tract or skin.

A better outlook for some

In some patients, however, the parts of the brain that have not been damaged can be expected to return to functioning more normally. The cells that remain alive in the damaged areas may start to work again within the first two weeks, and clinical improvement will then begin.

4 Clinical features of a stroke

If a doctor sees you within an hour or so of suffering what was probably a stroke, it may be difficult for him or her to be sure whether there is going to be minor or major damage so you will probably be admitted to hospital.

After 24 hours

Twenty four hours later, a number of patients will be completely better with no obvious, continuing problems and are diagnosed as having had a transient cerebral ischaemic attack. Most patients with a transient ischaemic attack have, however, recovered within a few minutes. They do require prompt assessment and investigation though, to detect and treat any underlying problem that could lead to a further attack, possibly more damaging than the first.

One week later . . .

After a week, many patients have made a good recovery and can be optimistic that the stroke will prove to be a minor one. If by two weeks, however, the patient is still severely troubled by speech disturbance, weakness, numbness, or a visual problem, the doctor can usually predict that there will be a considerable loss of function and the patient will probably need to stay in hospital for possibly two to three months.

What caused the stroke?

From the medical history and physical examination of the patient it is possible to say, in a proportion of cases, whether the cause was a cerebral infarct or a cerebral haemorrhage. Cerebral haemorrhages tend to come on very suddenly. The

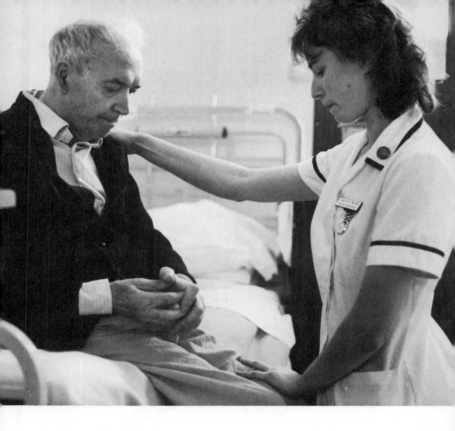

patient often has a severe headache at the beginning and sometimes vomits and loses consciousness. These symptoms are unusual, however, in cerebral thrombosis, where there is often a gradual increase in disability over a few hours. In someone who has suffered a cerebral embolism, the disability again occurs very suddenly but there may be clinical clues of embolism, such as an abnormal heart rhythm or heart murmur. Sometimes, the doctor cannot tell exactly what sort of stroke you have suffered when he examines you and thorough investigations are especially necessary.

Understanding the problem

The rest of this chapter deals with physical findings in stroke and should help patients who have suffered stroke or their relatives to understand the types of disability that arise.

Consciousness level

It is unusual for a stroke in the cerebral hemisphere to cause unconsciousness at the beginning, but patients who have had a very severe stroke affecting this part of the brain may start to become drowsy as cerebral swelling develops. Distortions occur inside the brain and the brain stem may be compressed, producing a gradual, progressive fall in consciousness. Most patients who have had a hemisphere stroke, however, remain conscious throughout.

Unconscious from the outset

If a patient is unconscious from the beginning a problem in the brain stem is likely because this is where the nerve cells concerned with being awake are located. Some patients never regain consciousness, but others tend to come round gradually over the first few days. A few patients are unconscious for a week or more and then recover, but the chance of recovery is reduced the longer a patient is unconscious.

Cerebral oedema

A 76 year old grandmother was found on the floor of her granny annexe when her daughter returned home from work. She was conscious but unable to say what had happened, was weak down the right side, and was unable to get up without assistance. The general practitioner was called and a hospital admission arranged.

When examined she was alert, had moderate weakness of the arm and a mild weakness of the leg. The next day, she was essentially the same but the day after that she became more drowsy, wouldn't or couldn't talk, and the arm weakness became severe. She remained in this state for three days and then started to improve – almost daily. Two weeks after the stroke she was able to feed herself and could just stand and walk a few steps with one assistant. At six weeks it was possible to allow her home. She still needed help bathing but could wash, dress, and feed herself and just walk without assistance.

Wide variation

The alertness of patients who are conscious varies considerably. Some may be fully aware of what is going on and sensible from the very start, and can immediately get on with the job of rehabilitation. Others are drowsy, disorientated, and generally confused and until this state of mind has improved there is little to be gained from attempts at rehabilitation.

Easily distracted

In the early days, most patients will have a poor attention span and will only be able to concentrate on things for a short period. They are readily distracted and because of this they may have a poor memory. In many cases, where there has been just one stroke, this tends to improve.

Weakness

When talking of strength and weakness, we tend to think immediately of the arms and legs but the muscles that control breathing and swallowing are much more important for survival and problems with these may be a major threat to life in the early days of a stroke. If the ability to swallow is severely affected, any fluids taken may get into the lungs rather than the stomach, causing choking and possibly pneumonia.

Poor swallowing

Swallowing is such a vital function that it is governed by nerves from *both* cerebral hemispheres. When one of the hemispheres has been affected by a major stroke, however, 'normal services' are temporarily disrupted and it may be 72 hours or so before the patient can swallow safely. During this time, the patient will need to be given necessary fluids via a tube into a vein (intravenous feeding) or by passing a tube through the nose and into the stomach (a naso-gastric tube). If the inability to swallow lasts beyond 72 hours, it is quite likely that the patient has had a previous problem affecting the other cerebral hemisphere.

Patterns of weakness

Often the face and arm on one side are moderately or severely paralysed and the leg on the same side is slightly less affected. This is the pattern of weakness when the stroke occurs in the territory of the middle cerebral artery. The middle cerebral artery is the continuation of the internal carotid artery and is therefore the most frequent site for a clot from the heart or major neck vessels to impact in the brain. Less frequently the patient's leg is much more severely paralysed than the arm and face on the same side and in this case it is usually the anterior cerebral artery that is involved.

Floppy limbs

To begin with the affected limbs tend to be floppy, with poor muscular tone and little in the way of movement at the hand, but some preservation of movement at the elbow and shoulder. The patient may be able to move the hip but fine movement of the toes or foot may be impossible.

Spasticity

As time passes, and by about two to three weeks, the reflexes return on the affected side and the muscle tone increases. The limb muscles usually develop an increased tone, which makes them stiff and is referred to as 'spasticity'. Don't be frightened or insulted by this term. In fact the spasticity that occurs in the muscles of the leg may be helpful (in moderation) because it may act as a form of internal splinting to make the leg more stable for standing and walking.

Walking

Most patients have a middle cerebral artery stroke and usually they will be able to walk. Their affected arm is often useful for holding objects, but the fine movements of the fingers and thumb may have gone and they may not be able to use cutlery or a pen in that hand. Patients with the less common variety of stroke, where the leg is more affected than the arm, may have difficulty returning to walking but may be able to use their hand quite well.

Speech

A severe problem with speech is something we all dread. Not to be able to understand what is going on or to communicate one's fears and needs is a horrifying prospect. Even simple requests like wanting to go to the toilet can be impossible to convey.

Talking

A problem in expressive speech will be obvious to everyone. If the patient is fortunate, there may only be a slight slurring of speech (as if drunk) as a result of paralysis of the side of the face and tongue. This dysarthria, as it is called, tends to recover reasonably well.

Damaged thought processes

More distressing problems occur where the thought processes concerned with the understanding and formulation of speech are damaged. Some patients may find it difficult to think of the right word and make mistakes which are irritating and only rarely amusing. Those who are more severely affected may be quite unable to say anything and others may just have one word like 'No', that they use for everything. Not only may the sufferer be unable to say what he wants, he may also be unable to write what he wants, in fact it is exceptional to find somebody who can write his needs clearly when he is unable to say them.

Therapy needed

A speech therapist is very valuable in this situation, not only for helping the patient, but also for helping the relatives to understand what the problems are and to help them communicate with their loved one.

Difficulty with understanding

Many patients with severe difficulties in expressing speech also have receptive problems so that they do not understand what

Jargon dysphasia

A 55 year old oil company executive had been to night school for navigation classes and got lost on his short journey home. In addition to being disorientated, his "stroke" involved a sudden difficulty in understanding spoken and written words. He seemed agitated and deranged and was taken to the local police station. Fortunately, someone realised he was ill and he was admitted to a psychiatric ward overnight. The problem with his speech was recognized and a neurologist was consulted. The man was transferred to the neurology unit for investigation. A brain scan showed that the problem was in the rear half of his dominant hemisphere, affecting the area responsible for receptive speech. His jargon dysphasia improved considerably but he did not recover sufficiently to return to his executive position.

is being said to them. This may be so severe that they are unable to understand simple commands like 'open your mouth', 'close your eyes' or 'touch my hand'. Having a stroke that has affected your speech is rather like waking up in a foreign hospital bed to find that you don't speak the language of any of the nurses or doctors and none of them speaks your language.

Sensitivity required

As with foreign languages, a patient's understanding tends to be better than the ability to speak. Medical staff and relatives must be extremely careful to avoid talking tactlessly in front of a patient after a stroke – just because stroke victims cannot talk, don't assume that they cannot understand. Much unhappiness is caused because people do not realise this and make tactless remarks in front of them.

Unwinspeek

Some patients will have a problem affecting their receptive speech more than their expressive speech, so that they are able to talk fairly well but it is badly 'monitored' by the brain and comes out as a form of nonsense or gobbledegook – the syle of speech (jargon dysphasia) assumed by the television comedian, Stanley Unwin.

It is quite possible for patients to have a stroke that affects their speech but does not cause any noticeable paralysis. The diagnosis of stroke may be missed in the early stages, particularly if the sufferer has jargon dysphasia, and an acute mental illness may be considered.

> **Just because stroke victims cannot talk, do not assume they cannot understand.**

Sensory disturbances

If a stroke has caused severe paralysis, the presence of a disturbance in feeling or sensation may not be fully appreciated by medical staff. The disturbed feelings may be relatively more serious than difficulties in the ability to detect a light touch, pinprick, and temperature. A severely affected patient may have considerable problems in interpreting what is happening on the affected side. They may have no idea where their limbs are in space without looking at them – in fact, they may have no feedback from the affected side at all. When someone draws their attention to the paralysed, insensitive limb, they may deny that it is anything to do with them and may even try to throw it out of bed using the good arm. This obviously makes rehabilitation much more difficult because the patient does not understand the problem, but fortunately these severe disturbances are rare. More commonly the patient has minor problems in knowing where his joints are, so that he is not quite sure where the hand or foot is and may have difficulty directing his arm into the sleeve of a jacket or his foot into a shoe. Often these sensations gradually recover with time, but sometimes disturbed skin sensations last and trouble the patient more than the weakness he is left with.

Pain

If a patient is particularly unfortunate and has a stroke affecting that part of the central grey matter of the cerebral hemisphere called the thalamus, he may suffer what is called the 'thalamic syndrome'. In this distressing condition sensations are distorted and the whole or part of the affected side feels painful. He may feel light touch or mild pressure as extreme pain and not unnaturally may attempt to avoid the bad side touching anything. Special drugs may be needed to reduce discomfort.

It's cold

After a stroke, patients may feel that their affected side is cold, and certainly it may be colder than the other side because of immobility. They should stimulate the cold hand and foot with the good side and wear warm clothing.

Prosopagnosia

A 65 year old housewife with high blood pressure and diabetes suffered a number of small strokes which did not cause any appreciable difficulty with balance, movement, or speech. One day however, she was looking out of the kitchen window and saw a strange man getting into her husband's car. She called the police saying that a man had stolen her husband's car, and they quickly found the car and stopped the driver, who turned out to be the husband. The woman was then examined by a doctor and was found to have a defect in recognizing familiar faces. She could, however, immediately recognize who it was when they spoke. To this day she can only make out who people are by using other clues like what they are wearing. She has lost the subtle ability of being able to put together the minor differences in facial appearance that allow her to recognize those who should be familiar to her, so every face seems strange!

Sight

In the early days after a stroke in the cerebral hemisphere, the patient's eyes may constantly look towards the good side. Unfortunately, this usually means that the stroke has been a severe one affecting more of the brain than just the area that controls the limbs. Eye deviation often means that the voluntary eye movement centre in the frontal lobe has been affected. Some patients whose vision is lost on one side because of damage to the relevant nerve pathways may also tend to look towards the good side, but their problems often resolve spontaneously.

Double vision

Patients with brain stem strokes will very often have the symptom of double vision and may occasionally feel that objects are moving and jumping. Fortunately these problems tend to be temporary.

Loss of vision

Patients can be reassured that they are not going to go blind when they find that they can't see properly after a stroke. Often, although vision is lost on one side, the patient has very little understanding of this fact because the part of the brain that lets him know that visual messages are going in (like the power-on light on electrical equipment) is also damaged. He may be quite content with what he can see in the remaining half of his visual field. As he gets better and starts to resume normal activities, however, he may find it quite unreasonable that he is banned from driving because of a defect that does not worry him at all.

Reading difficulties

If the left visual field is lost, patients will have difficulty finding the start of the next line when attempting to read and if the right field is defective they may find it difficult to know when they have reached the end of a line, especially in magazines and newspapers. A strip of coloured card placed vertically at the left or right side of a column of print may help. Books tend to be easier to read than newspapers and magazines with narrow columns, but in the early days patients have a poor attention span and may not be able to read for many minutes. Advice from a speech therapist may be helpful.

If the field defect is still severe after two weeks, recovery is unlikely to occur, but patients learn to cope with it better and when they return home and know the lay-out of furniture well, they are less likely to bump into objects on their 'blind side'.

Problems with interpretation

In addition to losing part of their visual field, patients may have considerable difficulty in interpreting what they see. They may be unable to recognise faces, even those of their spouse or family – and they may even be unable to recognise their own face in the mirror. Patients may have great difficulty finding objects in a room or drawer or working out what they are looking at when only part of an object is in view – for example, the handle of a knife, the corner of a book, or the toe of a shoe.

Other possible problems

Unfortunately, it is not only problems with speech, sight, and sensation that can occur – patients may find it difficult to remember things or to cope with fairly simple, everyday matters.

Memory

Memory problems may simply be caused by poor attention in the early days after a stroke and it is usually said that a stroke on one side does not produce a permanent memory defect. The memory stores are in the temporal lobes in *both* cerebral hemispheres and a permanent defect in memory usually means the patient has had more than one stroke in more than one cerebral hemisphere. The severity of a memory defect may vary considerably between people: some may be able to cope quite adequately with normal day to day activities whereas others are severely handicapped and need fairly constant supervision. Unfortunately, a series of strokes – not necessarily large, paralysing ones – may result in dementia, and it is therefore important to recognise a stroke when it occurs and take steps to prevent further attacks.

Memory problems in the early days may be caused by poor attention.

The apraxias

Although adequate movement and sensory function remain, some patients cannot 'put it all together' to perform even simple tasks. They may find it difficult to walk (walking apraxia), to dress (dressing apraxia), or to feed themselves and some may forget what is involved in going to and from the toilet. Treatment of these problems needs the skilled assistance of an occupational therapist and physiotherapist, and in most sufferers, some return of satisfactory function can be achieved.

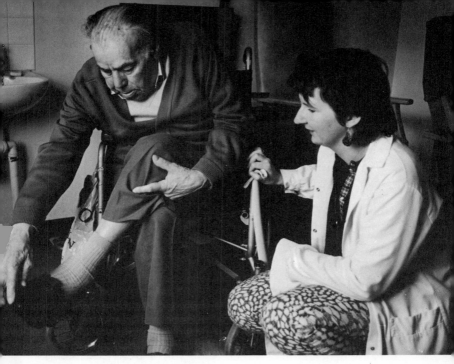

Apraxia — difficulty in dressing.

Continence

In the early days after a moderate or severe stroke, the patient may be unable to control his bladder or bowels but in most cases adequate control will be achieved eventually. In the immediate aftermath of a stroke the doctor may insert a fine tube into the bladder to drain it (urinary catheter). In practically everybody except the very old or those who have been unlucky and have had a stroke affecting areas of the frontal lobes specifically concerned with bladder control, the catheter can be removed. If a catheter has to stay, however, it can be made unobtrusive by using a leg bag that can be well hidden under trousers or a skirt. A patient with a catheter is at some risk from urinary tract infections and may need antibiotics, both for any infections that occur and, in some cases, in the long term to reduce the risk of reinfection. Patients with this problem need to drink a lot of fluids to reduce the chance of reinfection.

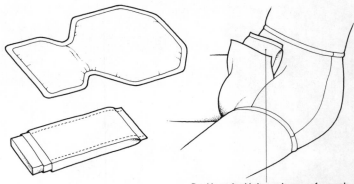

Incontinence aids.

Pad inserted into waterproof pouch

Regular toileting

Most patients with continence problems can be managed by regular toileting during the day and where necessary an absorbent pad or an external appliance can be used at night. Permanent loss of bowel control is very unusual and occurs in less than 10% of stroke victims.

5 Common complications after a stroke

Some people develop additional physical and emotional problems after they have suffered a stroke and we shall look at these in this chapter.

Frozen shoulder

Unfortunately, some stroke patients develop a painful, stiff shoulder on the affected side. There are three common causes for this. Firstly, the shoulder joint needs a full range of movement most days to keep it 'well oiled'. If this does not happen severe pain may be felt when the shoulder is moved. Secondly, a paralysed arm is very heavy and if left unsupported, will drag on the shoulder joint causing swelling and a painful, stiff joint. The third common cause of frozen shoulder is damage from the patient being lifted awkwardly under the armpit – part of the joint may be wrenched and inflamed as a result. Sometimes, even with the most careful nursing the patient develops a frozen shoulder and may need treatment with injections of local anaesthetics and steroids and physiotherapy to improve the power and range of shoulder movement. In most cases, satisfactory recovery occurs, but until it does, the shoulder causes pain both with movement and when lying on it.

Pneumonia

Because of poor swallowing and mobility and poor cough and lung expansion after a stroke, chest infections and sometimes pneumonia may occur. These usually respond to antibiotics and physiotherapy to improve lung expansion and remove phlegm. Occasionally, however, patients die, especially the elderly ones.

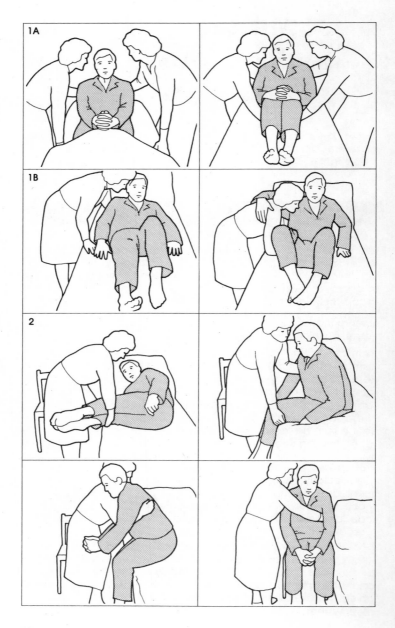

Lifting and moving (diagram opposite).

1A Lifting a stroke patient with two people
1B Lifting a stroke patient alone
2 Getting a stroke patient out of bed

Deep vein thrombosis and pulmonary emboli

It is extremely common for a thrombus, or clot, to form in the veins of the paralysed leg, especially in the calf. This may produce just a slight swelling of the ankle on that side with some tenderness in the calf, but sometimes the whole of the leg becomes swollen and uncomfortable. Because of the extra weight from fluid in the leg, movement is inhibited. Very occasionally the thrombus from the top-most part of the vein will break off to form an embolus which may find its way to the lungs blocking one or more of the pulmonary arteries which serve the lungs. This produces the disorder 'pulmonary embolism' in which there may be some chest pain and shortness of breath. Pulmonary embolism may occasionally be life threatening after a stroke, and is the cause of death in a small number of people.

Bed sores

Because the patient is paralysed and cannot feel, bed sores, particularly on the bottom, hips, ankles, heels, and even on the ear are a constant threat. But they are much more likely to occur in those who are diabetic or have lost bladder control. In an ideal world frequent turning and attention to the pressure areas would mean that patients never had bed sores. Unfortunately, they are seen not infrequently – even, occasionally, in the better hospitals with adequate nursing support! As well as being painful, bed sores represent a threat of infection – when the skin's surface is broken, 'germs' can get in. If a patient who has been immobile for many months gets an infection they may die.

41

Convulsions

A few stroke patients may have a fit or two in the early days after the attack, usually on the first or second day. In this there may be twitching and spasms of the muscles, noisy breathing, tongue biting, frothing of the mouth, incontinence, and loss of consciousness for a short time. These attacks are more likely to occur if the cerebral cortex itself has been affected, rather than deeper structures in the brain, and if the stroke has been caused by a cerebral embolism rather than a cerebral thrombosis or haemorrhage. Fits generally get better on their own and if not, they usually respond very well to anticonvulsant drugs. Most patients and relatives need not worry that fits will be a troublesome, continuing problem.

Emotional problems

People often feel depressed after a stroke. As well as the understandably low feelings that they have as an emotional reaction to such a sudden deterioration in the quality of their existence (reactive depression), many also suffer a physical or 'chemical' depression (endogenous depression). Depression is a common reason for patients failing to respond at the normal rate to attempts at remobilisation. Antidepressant drugs and a lot of understanding are often needed to lighten the mood and increase the patient's desire to cooperate with attempts at getting him better.

Spouses affected too

If the outlook for recovery is poor the spouse of the patient with stroke is also at risk from depression and changes in mood. There is always a major impact on the quality of his or her own future life and if the patient is dysphasic, this is particularly hard to bear. Husbands and wives of stroke victims may need counselling and antidepressant drugs to help them cope with their changed life.

Anger and resentment

In addition to depression, patients may feel angry and resentful and they often direct these feelings against the doctors and nurses who are caring for them. Relatively minor problems are often blown-up out of proportion and complaints are made. If this 'natural reaction' is understood by both the relatives and staff, any breakdown in communication that sometimes occurs can be prevented – to the benefit of all.

Altered personality

Some people seem to have a change of personality after a stroke. Their husband or wife will sometimes say, 'This isn't the person I married!' Quite often patients lack motivation, particularly if part of the frontal lobe is damaged, and this may limit their potential for recovery. Alternatively, they may become irritable, resentful, and very difficult to live with. The best way of coping with these changes is for the patient, his relatives, and the hospital staff to bring the problem out into the open by

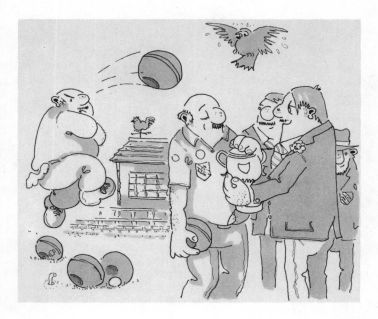

talking about it frankly. There is often a reluctance to do this, however, and a stressful situation may be made almost unbearable as a result. Fortunately, though, most patients are able to return to a quality of life that is satisfying, albeit more restricted than before. Joining self help groups and local clubs for stroke sufferers does much to improve mood and morale and also gives the carer a break for a few hours. Longer breaks for the carer by readmitting the more severely handicapped patients to hospital for a week or two every few months, can be arranged by the GP and local consultant.

Self-help groups do much to help morale.

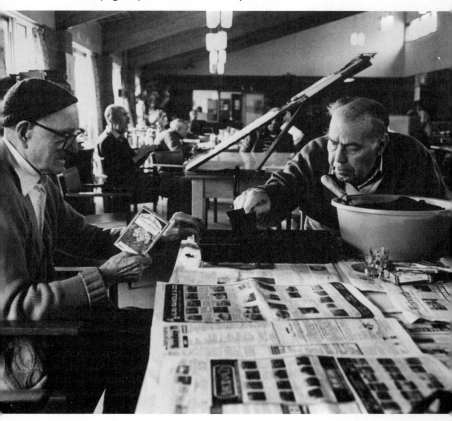

6 Tests and investigations

Doctors will do tests and investigations on a patient who has had a stroke. There are four main things they want to look at:

- The brain structure itself;
- The blood;
- The major arteries in the neck and the brain;
- The heart.

The brain

A special x-ray called a computed tomogram or another recently developed technique – nuclear magnetic resonance imaging – enable the doctor to 'look inside' the brain and help him determine what kind of stroke the patient has had. In this way a cerebral infarct can be distinguished immediately from a cerebral haemorrhage. These investigations have to be done reasonably soon after the stroke, however. If the patient is scanned over a month from the time of a haemorrhage – all the signs may have gone and the doctor cannot be sure if the stroke was caused by a haemorrhage or a thrombosis. Sometimes people have had more than one stroke, some of them cerebral infarcts and others haemorrhages, and it is important that this is recognised. A patient who has had a cerebral haemorrhage should not be given anticoagulation or antiplatelet drugs as these promote bleeding. Different forms of effective treatment may be needed for the two different conditions – thinning the blood for one but not the other – so an accurate diagnosis is of major importance.

Where and how big?

The location and extent of the haemorrhage or infarct, shown by the special x-rays can tell the doctor a great deal about the original cause. In a cerebral infarct, for example, it is sometimes possible to say whether the damage was the result of a cerebral thrombosis or an embolism from elsewhere. Furthermore, a computed tomogram of the brain will show

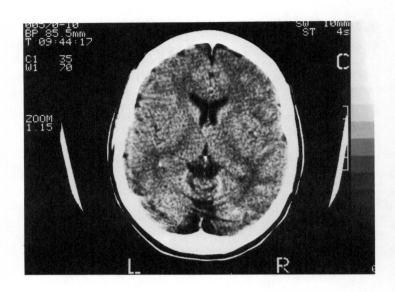

Computed tomograms of normal brain (above) and brain damaged by a stroke (below).

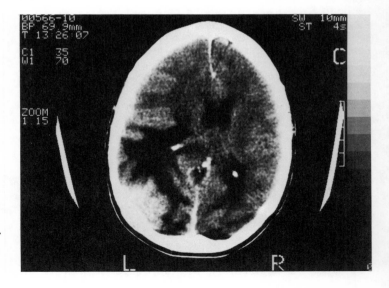

evidence of any previous trouble that may have occurred in the other hemisphere or in a different part of the same hemisphere, that was not obvious from the patient's medical history. This is important as approximately 50% of patients with stroke have some disturbance of speech, which limits their ability to give the doctor a full account of the event. The computed tomogram will show the amount of swelling and any shift or displacement of the various parts of the brain. It will also allow the doctor to see whether the cause of the stroke was a less common one, like a subdural haematoma or a subarachnoid haemorrhage. Finally, in a few patients who seem to have suffered a typical stroke, a scan will show a brain tumour.

Limitations of computed tomography

The computed tomogram fails to show a cerebral infarct in a minority of patients who have suffered one. This is because the scanner looks at the differences in the density of brain structures, and at the time of scanning the infarct and surrounding brain tissue may all be of the same density. In these patients, nuclear magnetic resonance scanning or another technique, positron emission scanning, may show up the abnormality.

The blood

Quite a number of blood tests will be needed for a full assessment. Firstly, the doctors will want to see if there are any disturbances of the blood that may have been directly responsible for the stroke itself. Secondly, they are used to determine if there are any other problems that may complicate the patient's recovery, such as a large reduction in body fluids (dehydration), disturbed kidney function, diabetes, or infection.

Blood disturbances

It is necessary to find out whether the patient's blood is too thick – that is, whether there is an increased concentration of the red blood cells. The examination of the white blood cells will give a clue as to whether there has been any recent infection that might have caused an increased tendency to clot... and therefore the stroke. Very occasionally, an unsuspected leukaemia or an abnormality of the platelets, or thrombocytes, will be found. Sometimes the results of a test called the sedimentation rate are high and this may mean that an inflammation of the arteries (an arteritis) rather than the usual narrowing of the arteries (arteriosclerosis) was the cause of the stroke.

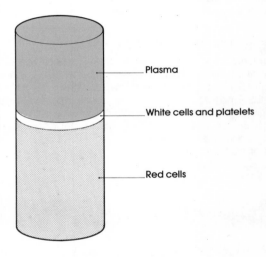

Plasma

White cells and platelets

Red cells

Main components of the blood.

Good management

To look after the patient properly, the doctor needs to know whether he or she is diabetic, whether the kidneys are working well (particularly in patients who are diabetic or who have high blood pressure), and whether their liver is working normally. Sometimes there is a clue pointing to alcoholism and the doctor can ensure that the added complication of an attack of delirium tremens (the DTs) caused by the sudden removal of alcohol can be avoided.

Investigation of the arteries

It should be emphasised that the main purpose of investigating the arteries is to see whether there is a problem that can be treated by surgery. It is not just to confirm that the patient has arteriosclerosis and to satisfy the doctor's curiosity!

Preventive not curative

Apart from a subdural haematoma, which can be easily seen on a computed tomogram, the two main problems that can be helped by operation are subarachnoid haemorrhage from a swollen leaking artery in the brain (aneurysm) or an appreciable narrowing in the neck part of the carotid artery (carotid stenosis). It should be emphasised that surgical treatment of the aneurysm and the carotid stenosis is to *prevent* further trouble – it cannot *improve* the rate or quality of recovery after an attack has already occurred. Indeed, if a patient is very poorly, investigation and surgical treatment need to be postponed, because there is a very high risk of surgery making a seriously ill patient worse. This reluctance to operate on patients who are sick and seem to need it most is sometimes difficult for relatives to understand.

Surgical treatment prevents further trouble. It cannot improve the rate of recovery after a stroke.

Non-invasive investigations

It is possible to get reasonable information on the state of the carotid and vertebral arteries in the neck using ultrasound techniques, and with newer machines really excellent pictures of the division of the carotid artery can be obtained. Ultrasound is less successful in showing the intracranial vessels, although it is now possible to tell whether the major arteries are actually open or not, and it is unsatisfactory in detecting aneurysm in the brain.

Angiography

In conventional angiography, a narrow, flexible tube (catheter) is inserted directly into the artery responsible for the stroke and a dye that shows up on x-rays is injected. In many hospitals, however, conventional angiography has given way to computerised digital angiography in which a vein in the arm is injected with the dye. This allows the doctor to see the abnormalities in the artery. In most cases sufficient information can be obtained simply this way rather than inserting a catheter. This newer technique runs only a very small chance of causing any complications and can provide very useful pictures of the carotid and vertebral arteries in both the neck and the brain.

Testing the circulation using ultrasound.

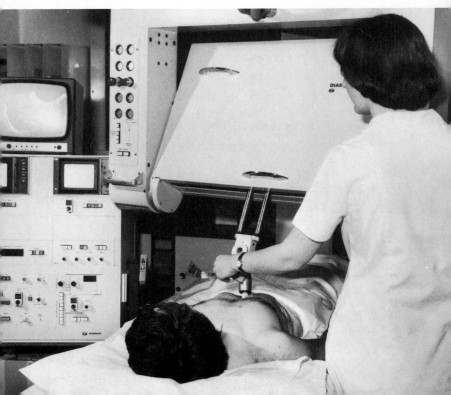

For precision – arterial digital angiography

If very precise pictures of the blood vessels in the brain are required, computerised digital angiography is still used, but the injection of dye is made through an extremely fine tube inserted into the aortic arch or neck arteries. This has only a very *small* chance of making the patient's condition worse provided he or she is in good general shape.

Aneurysm

Arterial digital angiography is used to detect an aneurysm in a cerebral artery. And the doctor can also use this technique to show the fine structure of the smaller blood vessels in the brain, if, for example, he suspects that an inflammation of the arteries, (an arteritis) was responsible for the stroke.

The heart

Every patient who has had a stroke needs to have a test called an electrocardiogram (ECG). This shows not only the rhythm of the heart beats, which is important as far as the development of blood clots is concerned, but also if there has been any recent or old heart attack (myocardial infarct).

A thrombus

If the doctor suspects that the stroke was caused by a blood clot from the heart another ultrasound technique, echocardiography, can be used. Echocardiography shows the chambers of the heart, the heart valves, the heart muscles, and the quality of heart contraction very precisely and it can also show evidence of a thrombus within the heart itself.

7 Treatment when a stroke occurs

For the moment, there is no miracle drug or operation that helps in the immediate aftermath of a stroke. Indeed many active treatments that, at first, looked hopeful have been shown to be positively harmful.

Current treatment for stroke aims:

- **To assist natural recovery;**
- **To prevent common complications (some patients are damaged further or even die as a result of complications that arise after stroke);**
- **To diagnose and treat promptly any complications that do occur.**

Breathing and swallowing

Management of these vital functions is a prime objective. The airway of a stroke patient who is unconscious may be partially obstructed as a result of a weak and paralysed tongue falling back and blocking the throat and difficulties with swallowing may cause an accumulation of saliva in the throat. Where these problems arise, the patient needs to be nursed on his or her side. Secretions often have to be removed by a suction tube and a plastic tube may have to be inserted through the mouth to provide a temporary airway. These patients need physiotherapy and they usually benefit from being given oxygen.

If the patient is going to survive, breathing usually recovers within the first few hours but swallowing difficulties may continue for a day or two, even in people who have had a first stroke. In those who have had more than one stroke, particularly if both sides have been affected, difficulty with swallowing may last for longer.

Fluid intake

Until natural recovery occurs, it is essential to maintain the patient's fluid intake by giving him liquid through either a fine tube into a vein (intravenous drip) or a tube from the nose into the stomach (naso-gastric tube).

Giving fluid into a vein.

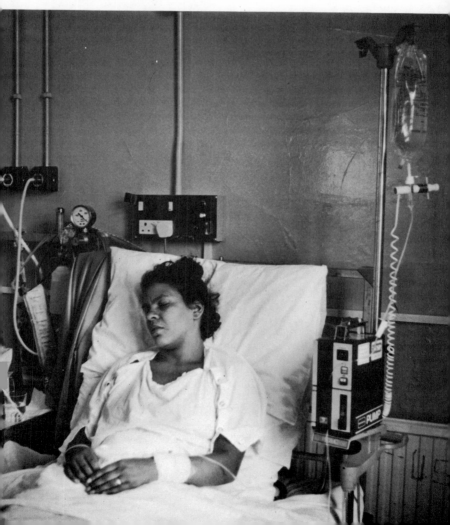

Convulsions

A few people who have had strokes may have a convulsion (fit) due to a sudden burst of electrical interference in the brain's normal electrical pattern. Convulsions need to be treated promptly to prevent further damage and anticonvulsant drugs like phenytoin and carbamazepine are usually given. It is only rarely necessary to continue these drugs in the long term.

Heart problems

Some patients, particularly the more elderly, may have mild heart failure at the time they have a stroke and this may become very much worse as a result of the stroke. The problem needs to be diagnosed early and treated with diuretic therapy (water pills) and drugs that improve the heart's efficiency, like digoxin. Any irregularity of the heart's rhythm will tend to reduce the output of blood from the heart and therefore threaten the blood flow to the brain so prompt recognition and treatment are required.

Deep vein thrombosis

It is extremely common for a blood clot or thrombus to develop in a vein in the paralysed leg. Many hospitals make patients wear special stockings in an attempt to reduce the chance of this complication and they also use a bed cradle to keep the sheets and blankets off the leg.

Treating deep vein thrombosis

When a deep vein thrombosis is detected, patients may need to go on to antiplatelet or anticoagulant therapy for a period of at least six weeks. Some doctors give all their patients a course of heparin (an anticoagulant) injected under the skin. This preventive treatment may limit the chance of developing a deep vein thrombosis without running the risk of bleeding from elsewhere.

Antiplatelet and anticoagulant therapy

Antiplatelet therapy is often prescribed for patients whose stroke has been shown to have been caused by a cerebral infarct rather than cerebral haemorrhage. They are given this treatment to prevent further trouble and to limit the spread of any blood clots in the arteries – anticoagulant therapy will not increase the rate of recovery from the stroke.

Anticoagulation immediately after a stroke

Anticoagulant therapy is now given relatively rarely to patients immediately after a stroke. When it was used in the past, a considerable number of patients bled from the damaged blood vessels in the region of the established stroke. There are, however, three situations in which anticoagulant therapy will be prescribed:

- Where a patient has had a number of transient cerebral ischaemic attacks that have tended to become longer and more severe despite antiplatelet treatment, and a computed tomogram shows no evidence of a haemorrhage. (This is known as *crescendo TIA*.)
- Where a stroke seems to be mild when the patient is first seen, but gradually increases in severity as time goes by. (This is known as a *stroke in evolution*.) Anticoagulation therapy probably benefits a proportion of these patients, but there is a risk of bleeding in others and it is not currently recommended in patients who are already considerably paralysed. A computed tomogram is also required to rule out any cerebral haemorrhage in these patients.
- When a patient has just had a stroke caused by a cerebral embolism from the heart, he or she runs a 15% risk of having a further embolism within the next two to three weeks. If a patient who has had a mild stroke is given anticoagulation therapy, this risk is reduced substantially. Where the stroke is moderate or large, however, immediate anticoagulation treatment may increase the risk of bleeding and is therefore not recommended. Patients who have suffered moderate damage as a result of an embolism may be considered for anticoagulation treatment two weeks after the first attack.

Many doctors do not consider that anticoagulation therapy is justified in patients with severe strokes.

Changes in the blood

The blood tests will show any blood disorders that may need to be corrected. Some patients' blood will be found to be very concentrated – with well over 50% being made up of cells. In most cases, this increased concentration of the blood is just caused by dehydration which leads to a reduction in the volume of plasma. Increasing the amount of body fluid by giving the patient fluid through a tube into a vein is all that is required. If the very high concentration persists, even after extra fluid has been given, however, some blood should be removed and replaced by clear fluid.

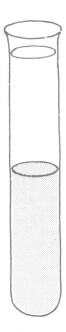

A question of dilution

There were some optimistic results from replacing blood with clear fluid (haemodilution) in patients whose concentrations of blood cells were reasonably normal but further studies have not confirmed the benefit. For the moment, only those with extremely 'thick' blood should be treated in this way.

Blood pressure problems

After a stroke it is normal to have an increase in blood pressure. This is partly due to an attempt by the body to keep the blood flowing to the brain at a time when the pressure within the skull has increased. In addition, when a main artery feeding the brain has been blocked, blood may reach the parts deprived of blood through a number of 'diversions' called collateral arteries and higher pressure is required to maintain an adequate blood flow through these.

Best left

The patient's blood pressure begins to return to normal within eight to ten days, and it is generally thought to be harmful to try to lower it within this period as blood flow to the vulnerable parts of the brain may fall to damagingly low levels as a result. Very occasionally, if a patient's blood pressure is dangerously high (at a level where it is going to increase the swelling in brain tissues, which in turn will raise the pressure within the skull even further), gentle, careful reduction is advised.

This contrast between the wish to treat high blood pressure in order to prevent a stroke, and to leave it alone afterwards is often misunderstood by relatives, who may become anxious about the blood pressure readings on the chart at the foot of the patient's bed.

Low pressure

If the patient's blood pressure is low after a stroke, it may mean that the normal reflexes governing blood flow are not working, and in this case the doctor may try to raise the blood pressure in order to improve blood flow to the brain.

Treating complications

Infections

Some patients develop chest infections and even pneumonia after a stroke. This is partly due to difficulties in coughing and removing salivary secretions and partly due to the poor breathing movement caused by paralysis of the chest on one side. Physiotherapy and antibiotic drugs are used at the first sign of trouble.

Bladder control

Patients often have difficulties with urinary control in the early days after a stroke. This can often be managed with frequent and regular toileting, but sometimes it is necessary to pass a flexible tube into the bladder, generally only for a period of a few days. Patients who regain their ability to control the passing of urine and stools within three to four days usually recover well. Some people develop a urinary infection at this time – even those who have not had a tube passed into the bladder – and so urine is tested regularly for signs of infection and treated with the appropriate antibiotic if necessary.

Keeping the temperature down

It is generally thought that it is harmful to allow a patient who has had a stroke to have a high temperature because the rate at which the brain cells have to work goes up with fever. Cells that are overworking in this way are thought to be more vulnerable when there is an inadequate supply of blood.

Surgical treatment

Surgery is only rarely helpful in the period immediately after a stroke, and it is felt that a general anaesthetic and the effects of surgery may well make matters very much worse. The main reason for this is that the brain's blood supply is normally preserved by highly responsive cerebral vessels that change in size as the need dictates, a phenomenon called auto-regulation. After a stroke, this ability to respond is temporarily lost and a fall in blood pressure during surgery may then cause further brain damage.

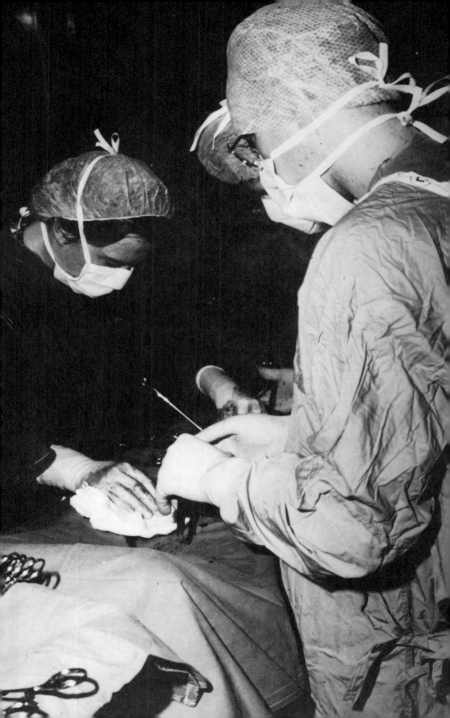

When is surgery needed?

Surgery may be needed to clear a rapidly expanding cerebral haemorrhage. This is particularly necessary in patients who have suffered a haemorrhage into the cerebellum. Here, the effects of a blood clot are felt very much more quickly and there may be a rapid rise in pressure within the skull causing compression of the brain stem. A patient with this problem may suffer a rapidly deteriorating level of consciousness. Removing the clot may be life saving in this situation and apart from difficulties with balance, patients can recover well.

In the cerebral hemisphere

Bleeding in the cerebral hemisphere should only be treated by surgery if it is very near the surface of the brain and is expanding and causing pressure symptoms. Pressure symptoms include increasing headache, vomiting, and a fall in the level of consciousness.

An aneurysm

Patients who have had a subarachnoid haemorrhage from a leaking Berry aneurysm or a defect in an artery or vein should be offered surgery, particularly if they make a good recovery from their first attack.

Thrombosis

The place of surgery after a stroke caused by thrombosis is really to prevent further trouble. Patients who have been shown to have narrowing in a carotid artery that was responsible for the stroke and who make a good recovery can be offered surgery to remove the thickened lining of the artery (carotid endarterectomy), which should help prevent further trouble.

Nursing care and other specialist therapies

Good nursing care is of paramount importance in the early days after a stroke, it can help prevent some of the complications outlined above and should also prevent the risk of developing pressure sores caused by lying in bed in one position (bed sores). Patients also benefit from physiotherapy at this time to keep their joints mobile and to prevent breathing problems and lung infections. Speech therapy soon after a stroke may help patients cope with swallowing difficulties and communication, and will also help the relatives understand about any problems. The aid of an occupational therapist is also required in order to assist the patient with feeding and early self care. The role of these therapists becomes more important after the first two weeks, however, when the patient has recovered from the physical shock of the stroke and needs rehabilitation therapy.

Morale

It is vital to keep the morale of the patient and his or her relatives going at this time. Appearances really matter – women should have their hair done and their face made up as before, and men should be shaved. Although false teeth can be a problem because of facial and cheek weakness on one side, denture adhesive may be helpful.

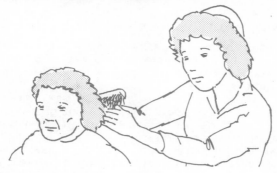

Maintaining morale

Maintaining the morale of patients who have had a mild stroke but whose recovery is obvious within the first few days is not difficult. But for more severely affected patients who show little or no sign of improvement and, in fact, a slight deterioration in the first week because of cerebral oedema, it is important to remember that in the first two weeks, there is a medical illness and the extent of any damage may be difficult to assess until the beginning of the third week.

Treatment of the future

It is likely that any effective, future treatment will need to be given promptly – within a few hours of the onset of a stroke – and this means that patients will have to be referred to hospital speedily. Then they will need urgent brain scanning investigations to determine whether the stroke has been caused by a cerebral haemorrhage or cerebral infarct. Those with infarcts, especially the younger patients, may need angiography, and then when the clot has been found, anticoagulation drugs will be introduced locally, using the same catheter as for the angiography. In the past, drugs have been given to stroke patients through a vein, but now this treatment has been abandoned because of subsequent bleeding problems. It is hoped that giving drugs directly to the part of the brain in greatest need will achieve good results with as few complications as possible.

Enzymes may help

Some of the chemical changes that occur in and around the damaged part of the brain prevent recovery, and removing these or stopping their effect may help both the rate and extent of improvement. Research has indicated that brain cells are more likely to survive if the blood flow stops altogether, rather than if a trickle of blood continues. All the brain needs to keep it working is adequate amounts of oxygen and glucose and removal of waste products. Both these functions are carried out by the circulatory system. Immediately after a stroke, when the circulation is not functioning and there is just a trickle of blood, the damaged areas are very short of oxygen but there is some glucose. The glucose cannot be broken down and used properly, however, and waste products are produced that cannot be removed. When blood flow is restored, there is an enormous inflow of oxygen and the brain may not be ready for it. Poisonous substances called free radicals may be formed as a result. Some enzymes, called catalase and dismutase, have been used in experiments and have been shown to produce a reduction in the poisonous, free radicals in brain tissue. This enzyme treatment may be tested in patients in the near future.

Minimising the damage

Laboratory work has shown that many brain cells can survive a deficiency of blood for longer than was previously believed. This gives hope that by removing a clot quickly or speeding the resorption of blood from a haemorrhage and then preventing the problems outlined above, the damage caused by a stroke will be reduced and the resulting handicap minimised.

Patient on life support machine.

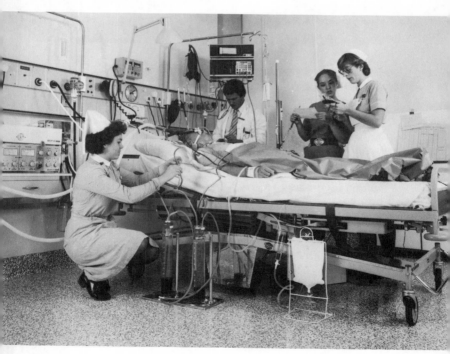

8 After the first two weeks

In many patients the physical illness of stroke is past at two weeks. Many patients will be improving daily. In others, however, serious paralysis or sensory change will persist and if they are left with some disability they will have to learn to cope with it.

Prospects

At this stage, the doctor should have a good idea of how recovery is going to proceed. When the patient's hand is affected, for example, but he can move his fingers and thumb at two weeks, the doctor can be optimistic that the hand will recover well. If there is no sign of finger movement and very limited movement at the shoulder and elbow, it is likely that the hand and arm may only be useful for steadying objects to be manipulated by the good hand. Only one in seven patients recovers the use of their arm if it has been paralysed. If there is some movement at the hip and knee, it is likely that the patient can be taught how to walk again but stroke victims who still cannot control their bladder at two weeks have a poor chance of walking.

Order of recovery

The order of recovery varies from one patient to the next. The table can be used, however, as an approximate guide for someone who has had a moderate to severe stroke.

Guide to recovery

- **Can control his or her bowels;**
- **Can sit in a chair without slumping or sliding out of it;**
- **Starts to attempt to feed him or herself with the good hand;**
- **Can control his or her bladder (there may be difficulty with patients whose speech has been affected, who may not be able to indicate that they need to go to the lavatory);**
- **Cooperates with good side on being moved;**
- **Stands better and starts to walk with two assistants.**
- **Attempts to wash, comb hair, shave with electric razor, and part-dress.**
- **Walks with one assistant, can usually get up alone;**
- **Walks independently, possibly with tripod or stick;**
- **Fairly independent at washing and feeding;**
- **Attempts stairs and is discharged home.**

Sensory problems

Recovery is always slower in patients who have serious sensory problems, and this is particularly so if their understanding of where their arms or legs are in space is faulty. The ability of the brain to interpret messages from the affected side may be so poor that the patient shows no interest in the paralysed side, and even neglects it. Rehabilitation of these patients can be particularly difficult.

After six months

Physical recovery is largely over by six months and is greatest during the first three months. The table illustrates the percentages of stroke victims who will not have recovered from a disability by six months. Any patient who cannot walk at six months will not be able to walk again.

Disability: percentage who will not have recovered by six months

- Unable to speak 10
- Still incontinent 10
- Needs some help washing 10
- Cannot walk alone 15
- Needs some help eating 20
- Needs some help with toileting 20
- Needs some help to transfer from bed to chair 20
- Needs some help with dressing and stairs 30
- Needs some help to bathe 50

Up to two years

Some further recovery can occur up to two years after the stroke. Thereafter, any improvement is usually the result of the patient having learnt some trick movements and not any actual improvement in the way their brain or nervous system is working. In rare instances, however, definite improvement continues over a longer period.

The challenge of looking after a patient with stroke is to cope with the disability, to achieve some improvement, and to prevent a further stroke.

Nursing care

In the more severely affected patients, nursing care is still of high priority for the first six to eight weeks. It is important to move the patient regularly to avoid bed sores, to position the patient appropriately, and to move the joints to avoid permanent stiffening.

Bladder and bowels

Any problems with the bladder and bowels need expert attention. It is usually possible to cope with difficulties over bladder and bowel control by regular toileting, particularly on waking, after meals, and at night, and only a minority of sufferers need a drainage tube in the bladder long term. Some patients, however, may need appliances such as incontinence pads at night. Problems with bowel control may be eased by keeping the patient slightly constipated and using a laxative or suppository every third day.

Physiotherapy

After two weeks, physiotherapists start to take a much more active role in helping recovery and they also try to prevent the patient developing bad habits. As patients improve, some muscle movements tend to recover more quickly than others. Bad posturing can result, and this hinders improved function in the long run. The ability of the muscles to contract increases, which may mean that they become so stiff they prevent full joint movement. Some exercises can be counter productive, though. Sometimes, for example, patients are given a rubber ball to squeeze in an attempt to improve their grip. In fact, the way to improve hand function is to teach the patient to straighten their fingers and wrist rather than bend and contract them because otherwise the hand develops an increasingly flexed posture and if left untreated the fingers may be so firmly turned into the palm it may be impossible to straighten them.

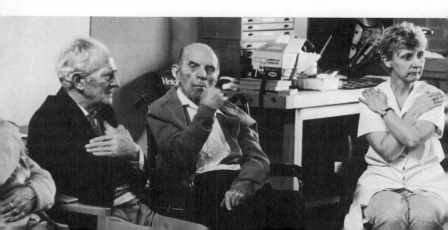

Balancing act

At first there is much emphasis on teaching patients to recover their sense of balance. It's a bit like a child learning to walk – he cannot stand before he can sit and he cannot walk before he can stand. Patients are taught to sit without support and to avoid the tendency to fall to one side. They then learn to stand and to walk with one or two helpers. Eventually, patients graduate to using a walking frame, then a tripod, then, hopefully, a stick and then, even more hopefully, alone. Sometimes a splint is required to support a dropped foot a weak knee or wrist.

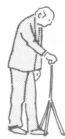

Get the family involved

It is important for relatives to get involved in rehabilitation, particularly as the time approaches for the patient to go home. They must learn how to help move, how to lift, and how to support the patient, particularly when walking.

It also helps if they know how to guide him through the exercises that reduce spasticity and improve movements so that he can continue to do these when he returns home. The physiotherapist cannot do the job without help and patients need their support and encouragement too.

Different approaches

Schools of phsyiotherapy differ in their approach to rehabilitation. Some now attempt to prevent the patient using his good side for intervals each day to reawaken his interest in the weak side and to overcome 'learned non-use'. This jargon phrase means that the brain, after discovering that the paralysed side is not doing what is required, gives up and concentrates on the good side. There are schools that put some emphasis on teaching the good side new tricks, for example eating one handed and writing with the left hand if you are right handed.

How can a physiotherapist help

A physiotherapist can help prevent complications like frozen shoulder, permanent joint stiffness, or pneumonia. She can explain and help to show patients how to overcome problems such as:

- How to turn over in bed (something we all take for granted);
- How to improve balance and to sit and stand again without toppling;
- How to walk;
- How to use a frame, tripod, or stick;
- How to cope with stairs.

Speech therapy

Speech therapists can help the patient and his or her family understand the exact nature of the communication problem – whether there is just a problem in expressive speech (rare), how much difficulty with understanding, reading, and writing there is. Patients often respond to gestures and to the emotional content of a conversation and may therefore understand less than you think initially and more than you think later. In the early days, the emphasis may be on non-verbal communication where the patient has a set of pictures on a board or card that he can point to, to indicate his basic needs. Relatives should be involved in the speech therapy sessions from the beginning so that they can continue the programme for recovery whenever they visit.

Aide memoire

Relatives and friends who want to help with the recovery programme need to remember the following points:

- Are any false teeth in and fitting? (some denture adhesive may be helpful);
- Is any hearing aid in and on?
- Are the patient spectacles on?
- Have they removed distractions? (Turn off the radio or television);
- Don't shout unless the patient is deaf;
- Short sessions only to begin with.

Most recover some speech

Most patients can be taught to recover sufficient speech to make their basic needs understood. But this may seem too much to hope for when only a few incomprehensible grunts can be achieved in the early days. The patient and his relatives may need frequent support to keep their morale high so that they persevere even when progress seems very slow.

Speech aids

Speech aids are disappointing in dysphasic patients and are almost never used. Simple typing devices may, however, be helpful for patients who fail to learn to write adequately again because of poor motor skills, but whose understanding of language is good.

Occupational therapy

The occupational therapist helps to teach the patient how to feed himself, wash, comb his hair, shave, dress, cope with the toilet, and eventually with the kitchen – a major landmark is when he can make a cup of tea himself. These therapists provide aids to help make eating and drinking easier and less messy.

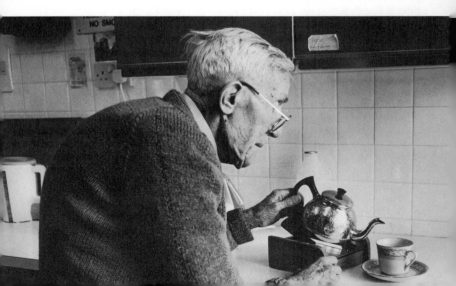

Using the hands

Occupational therapists are particularly concerned with reha-bilitating the hands, if necessary teaching patients how to cope with just one good hand. One handed shoe laces are available and modifications to clothing using Velcro rather than zips or other fasteners may be necessary.

Assessing the patient's home

Sometimes before discharge home is planned, the hospital occupational therapist and the district occupational therapist will arrange a visit to the patient's home to assess what modifications and aids will be needed. It is usually necessary to provide a number of aids including a commode, special rails on the stairs and corridors, and grips in the bathroom and in the toilet. A bath stool and bath mat are usually necessary.

Modifications

Even relatively minor disabilities require some modifications to the home to increase the patient's potential activities and independence. A bed may need to be brought downstairs, or a stair-lift installed. Nursing a patient with one-sided weakness in a double bed is difficult, and in most cases he will have to start off in a single bed. Furniture may need to be rearranged so that the room is not cluttered or dangerous, and loose rugs should be removed. Suitable well fitting shoes with a good grip should be worn not loose slippers!

Mobility aids

The occupational therapist will also arrange for walking frames and wheelchairs for home use if necessary. The therapist is often reluctant to suggest a wheelchair and the patient may be unwilling to accept one. The obvious wish is to avoid reliance on a wheelchair and to encourage patients to attempt to walk and be more independent. Sometimes, however, a wheelchair can widen the stroke victim's horizons – allow him or her to go shopping, to get about more, and improve morale generally. Eventually, the occupational thera-pist may be helpful in arranging for the car to be modified so that the disabled person can drive.

Medical social worker

Stroke is such a bombshell, that the victim and his family are very often caught completely unawares. They may need help and advice on things like employment and domestic and financial problems (both in the short and long term) in hospital and on returning home. Sometimes, for example, if a husband is paralysed and dysphasic and there are no joint bank accounts, his wife may be completely unable to get any money. A medical social worker will help the family to cope with this, she will also advise on the state benefits that are available and to which the patient is entitled, both in hospital and afterwards.(See the list of DHSS leaflets at the end of the book.)

Power of attorney

If the stroke sufferer is unable to look after his own financial affairs, it may be necessary to enrol the help of a solicitor and to obtain 'power of attorney'. Citizen's advice bureaux should be able to advise on this.

Rehabilitation units

In the early weeks, stroke patients may have relatively poor stamina and cannot take long periods of remedial therapy. After four to six weeks, however, depending on the severity of the stroke, they (and their relatives) often start to complain that they are not getting enough help. The stage has been reached where they can cope with longer periods of activity and they may feel that they are not getting enough attention as more acutely ill patients are admitted to the ward. It is understandable for the nursing and medical staff to pay more attention towards a new, perhaps unknown problem rather than the well established and stable one.

Patients should be transferred

Ideally, patients who have reached this stage should be transferred to a rehabilitation unit where they can have physiotherapy, occupational therapy, and speech therapy for several hours each day. In these units, where people are getting better and more mobile, the morale is often high. They have a different atmosphere from hospital and certainly patients are spared the trauma of other inmates suddenly dying or developing distressing problems.

Units are expensive

The units are very expensive, however, as there is a high number of staff in relation to patients, and they are not widely available around the country. It is a sad reflection on the facilities available that most stroke patients do not have the benefit of a specialised rehabilitation unit. As rehabilitation units increase the rate of recovery and speed the patients' return home there is a considerable saving on bed costs. Those unable to benefit from one, however, should take comfort from the fact that by the end of a year there is probably little difference in their achievement and that of someone who has been to a rehabilitation unit.

Most patients go home

The vast majority of stroke patients do eventually get home. Only a small proportion need permanent care in a hospital or residential home and they tend to be the very elderly or those who had physical or mental problems before they suffered a stroke. A patient who already had dementia for example, would achieve little improvement after a stroke. The relatives of patients who cannot return home should find a satisfactory nursing home with the help of the social worker. Only occasionally will it be necessary for a stroke patient to stay in a hospital in the long term.

9 Going home

Attitudes to returning home differ widely. Some patients want to go home far too soon and if allowed to do so may meet difficulties that they and their family could have been spared. As a result, they may become very demoralised. Others, however, are surprisingly reluctant to leave the protected environment of hospital, even when they are ready to do so. They worry about facing the risks of the outside world without support and help from the doctors, nurses, and other therapists which they have come to expect in hospital. One day the plunge has to be taken, however, and patients almost always cope very much better than they thought they would.

But support is needed

It is nearly always possible to let a patient return home if their husband or wife is still alive and able to care for them. Widowed or single people may be able to go home if support is available from children or other family members, but it must be remembered that married children are often in a genuinely poor position to help. They may have a demanding young family, they may be out at work all day and unable to afford to stop, or they may live in a flat or house that is too small to accommodate an infirm relative. Approximately 30% of old people have no close relative to rely on for support after a stroke and many of these will need to be looked after in a nursing home rather than returning to their own home.

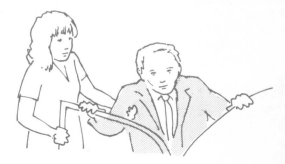

Improving facilities at home

Before a stroke patient is allowed home from hospital, steps should be taken to improve home facilities and support. Apart from the modifications and aids mentioned earlier on p. 71, other more complicated pieces of apparatus may become necessary. Things like automatic page turners for newspapers or books may be needed or devices that allow handicapped people to turn lights, televisions, and radios on or off. Remote control television and music apparatus may also be a great boon. It will not be long before robots will be available for helping handicapped people at home. They are already at the planning stage!

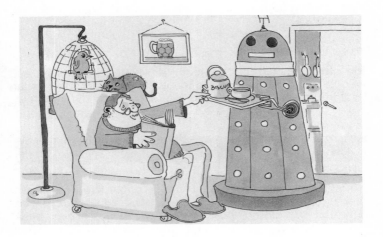

The GP takes over

After discharge from hospital the general practitioner takes over responsibility from the hospital consultant, although it is quite common for the patient to see the hospital physician again if further advice is required. It is also common for a single outpatient appointment to be made after discharge to check that all is going well. Outpatient appointments for further speech therapy and physiotherapy may also be necessary.

Organising support

Some of the support services available are organised through the general practitioner. District nurses may be necessary to help with bathing the patient, to apply dressings, or to help with control of the bowel. A home help is often arranged and may prove to be of great value. Some patients or their carers resist the suggestion of help because of a wish to be independent, but they should be advised to at least give it a try. Meals on wheels may also be a great boon.

Attendance allowance

The attendance allowance from the Department of Health and Social Security that many stroke patients are entitled to allows the victim's spouse to hire further help to give her some time off, even if this means just enough time to go shopping or to the hairdressers.

Clubs and groups

The patient should join the local 'stroke club' or similar 'self-help' group. Failing this, it is often possible to arrange regular visits to a hospital day unit. Getting out is essential for morale.

Diet

Although most people worry about cholesterol, the main problem to face in someone who is physically handicapped after a stroke is an increase in weight due to lack of exercise. A vicious circle can occur, where an increase in weight makes the patient more immobile and so that he puts on even more weight and becomes even more immobile. In addition, the extra weight will make it increasingly difficult for the carer to move or lift the patient.

The answer to being overweight is to eat less, to have small regular meals, and to be as active as possible.

Reducing fat intake?

By all means reduce the fat intake, it will help patients to lose weight, but for most people over 50, there is probably very little benefit to be gained from low fat diets unless the doctor has confirmed that there is a medical reason for this. Restriction of carbohydrates is particularly necessary if the patient is diabetic and will help to minimise weight gain.

Avoiding constipation

Another challenge is to avoid the constipation that is common in people who cannot move around well. The diet should be high in roughage – brown bread, breakfast cereals containing bran, fruit and vegetables. Sometimes medicine is required, for example lactulose (Duphalac), sterculia (Normacol), ispaghula husk (Regulan or Fybogel), and many handicapped patients are helped by glycerine suppositories every third day. It is not necessary to have a bowel action everyday and strong laxatives should be reserved for emergencies only.

Alcohol

Alcohol consumption should be reduced to a maximum of three units a day (three single measures of spirits or one and a half pints of beer). Some patients may find that even one unit will make it even more difficult to cope with their disability, whereas others may be helped by small amounts.

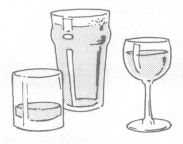

Remember many men put on weight from what they drink and not from what they eat, and with the current cost of alcoholic drinks many of us have very expensive 'spare tyres' indeed!

Medication

Patients will usually be given a supply of tablets for a few days after leaving hospital and this will be renewed by their general practitioner (but do remember to call him). The common medications prescribed are those for treating high blood pressure and heart problems like irregularity of heart rhythm and minor heart failure.

Other drugs

A number of patients will be given antiplatelet therapy in the form of aspirin or dipyridamole, or both, in an attempt to prevent further clots forming, not only in the blood vessels in the brain but also in the heart. Some patients will require insulin tablets or injections for diabetes, others may need anti-depressant or anticonvulsant drugs.

Stop unnecessary drugs

The medication should be reassessed from time to time and any unnecessary drugs should be stopped. Patients often need sleeping pills when they are in a noisy hospital ward, but they should try to do without them once they have settled in again at home. Remember that people can become more depressed through using sleeping pills regularly and the sedative effects of these drugs often lasts well into the next day.

Emotional problems

Although some patients feel much happier when they get home, emotional problems may become very much more obvious after discharge from hospital. Relatives may be surprised by the depth of the depression which they had missed or misinterpreted during the relatively short hospital visiting periods each day. Antidepressant drugs may be necessary for a month or two and most people respond well to these but occasionally stroke patients need help from a psychiatrist.

Extreme anxieties

Some patients may be afraid to go out – known as agoraphobia. They may be embarrassed at meeting other people, even old friends, because of their speech defect and physical disability. They may become self conscious about appearance or perhaps anxious about getting to the toilet in time.

Depression

A 55 year old car mechanic who had high blood pressure found it impossible to give up smoking. He had been under much pressure at work and had been overdoing things for some months. He woke one morning, was able to get to the bathroom but while shaving dropped his razor and was unable to return to the bedroom. His wife found him slumped on the floor. He was admitted to hospital and found to have a mild to moderate right-sided weakness with some difficulty expressing himself. He had good appreciation of where his limbs were in space and the outlook for recovery and regaining independence was predicted to be good. However, he failed to make the expected recovery. The therapists felt that he was not interested and seemed to have no motivation. It was suspected that he was depressed, although exact confirmation of this was not easy because of his speech defect. He was started on an antidepressants and within a week improvement began. A month after returning home, it was possible to stop the antidepressants without any evidence of a relapse.

Boredom

Staying at home all day with little to do except watching television may produce a profound boredom. This is particularly troublesome if the spouse is working and the patient has to be left at home for long intervals, more or less on his own. The sufferer may be very frustrated by his or her disability and become irritable and very negative as a result. These problems should be spotted early and talked over with the general practitioner who may arrange for them to visit a stroke group or day centre, if he or she is not already doing this.

Some of the emotional problems are triggered by underlying intellectual changes. Unfortunately patients do sometimes change in that they develop a lack of insight into their disability and mood. They lack drive and motivation, which often causes conflict with the family, criticism, resentment, arguments, and a further reduction in contact with others. Counselling from one of the team of professional contacts may be both necessary and helpful for both sufferers and their families.

Intellectual difficulties

These again may only become very obvious to the family on the patient's return home and sometimes they are not spotted until the patient returns to work. Even patients without any obvious speech defect may have problems organising their thoughts and planning the simplest of tasks. They may also have a lack of understanding and recognition and lack of foresight. Someone who has had a stroke may be quite unable to do simple arithmetic, which makes it difficult for them to go shopping and impossible to cope with change. They may be unable to help to make the family decisions and, in some cases, this means the spouse has to take on a new role as the dominant partner. Even relatively minor intellectual defects, which interfere little with the day to day life at home, may make a return to work impossible.

Denial

A 70 year old, right handed nun suffered a stroke in the back half of the right cerebral hemisphere, which caused difficulty with vision on the left side and disturbed feeling on the left side of the face, hand, and leg. She had no idea where her arms and legs were in space — they did not feel as if they belonged to her. She got extremely agitated that there was someone else in bed with her and made attempts to throw the left side of her body out of bed. This resulted in a number of falls and bruises despite the nurses' attempts to prevent her damaging herself. Although this very disturbing collection of sensations cleared within two to three weeks, very considerable problems persisted and we were not able to get her to use the right hand or to walk. Fortunately, the order she belonged to was able to look after her despite these disabilities and she seemed to enjoy herself — her intellectual interests remained and she was able to hold a good conversation.

Resuming contact with others

Close relatives and friends may well have visited while the patient was in hospital and it is important to keep this up once he has returned home. The patient should spend much of his time in the heart of the family, not in the spare room, and he should feel included in any conversation. Plenty of contact with others usually helps to overcome agorophobia and encourages the patient to leave home and visit others. Many sufferers resist the idea of going out and make all sorts of excuses to avoid this, so support and reassurance from the doctor or district nurse are often necessary before they will agree to leave home. It is only too easy to understand why some sufferers don't want others to see their paralysis, difficulty walking, or speech disturbance.

Dysphasic people need to feel 'included' emotionally. If you are in a group, sit by them, put your hand on theirs, turn towards them, refer to them, and use gestures so that they are not set apart.

Returning to work

Only a small proportion (approximately 15%) of patients who are working at the time of their stroke ever get back to full time employment. This is partly because many working people who have a stroke are nearing retirement age and many accept early retirement on health grounds. Remember that the advice of the medical social worker may be very helpful here to sort out what can be a very complex situation and to ensure that you achieve the best financial deal.

Speech defects cause most problems

Patients with speech disturbance have the greatest problems in returning to work. Those who are left with any speech defect almost always find it difficult, if not impossible, to cope with any sort of administrative post. Those with physical disability will obviously find it very difficult to resume any manual or skilled employment.

Large companies are more flexible

People who have been employed by a large company have a better chance of being accepted back at work as other jobs that are within their intellectual and physical capabilities can often be found. Small companies cannot be so flexible and it may be quite impossible to cope with a previous job unless fully fit.

Some have triumphed

There have, however, been some notable triumphs in people returning to work after stroke. Perhaps the greatest and best known of these is the scientist Louis Pasteur, who continued to do remarkable original work of great scientific importance for many years after his severe stroke.

Back into the driving seat

Patients who have made a good recovery after a stroke may approach the Driver and Vehicle Licensing Centre (DVLC) in Swansea after six months to discuss the question of driving. After a transient ischaemic attack, the period is three months, but if the patient has had more than one transient ischaemic attack, he or she needs to wait six months from the last attack.

Fit to drive?

The DVLC will normally allow a stroke victim to drive if they have no significant motor, sensory, or visual defect that makes it difficult or dangerous for them to be in control of a motor vehicle. The doctor and the patient's relatives should also be happy that he or she has sufficient judgement to be able to drive. Demented patients may prove difficult to dissuade from driving, which can be tricky for carers. The medical advisers to the DVLC may well suggest that the patient has a licence for just 12 months in the first instance.

Assessing capabilities

In cases of doubt, when the doctor feels that the patient's disabilities may well be getting in the way of his ability to control a car, an assessment should be made of his perform-ance behind the wheel. The British School of Motoring run a number of disabled driver assessment units and the patient should be referred to one of these and should agree to be bound by their verdict.

Modifying the car

It is often necessary to modify the car. One with automatic transmission is very much easier to drive than a car with manual gear change and in some cases it may be necessary to convert the car to hand controls.

Convulsions

A patient who has had a convulsion after his or her stroke will not be allowed to drive for 12 months, and if he has had more than one convulsion, the DVLC insist on an observation period of two years from the *last* attack.

Insurance

The insurance company should be informed of the stroke and plans to resume driving. They will usually require a letter from the doctor or specialist supporting these plans. Insurance premiums are often increased a little but if the company is not informed of the stroke the insurance may be nul and void.

Sex after stroke

For most stroke victims there is no reason why sex should be abandoned. Sexual intercourse does not increase the risk of having another stroke. Having said this, however, a change in roles may be necessary to accommodate any physical disabilities and there may be emotional problems that need to be overcome. Dr Christine Sandford's book *Enjoy Sex in the Middle Years* (published by M Dunitz Ltd) is helpful reading.

Conclusion

The quality of life after a stroke may be surprisingly good despite some remaining disability. Patients will often say that they had not realised how much of a rut they were in, slaves to the work routine, never taking time to enjoy other aspects of life. Some people become quite outward-going and have a new lease of life. This is much easier with a supportive spouse and family, but it can also be achieved in the better run nursing homes where there is good morale and plenty going on.

10 Carers need care too

Your relief that your relative has survived may conflict with your worries and fears about the future. People often say, 'How will I manage?' 'I don't think I will be able to cope.'

Let others help

Some voluntary organisations (see p. 104) and a handful of local authorities run courses to help carers. You must accept as much help and support as you can, both at home and outside it. At home, you can have assistance from a home help, district nurse (or nurse aid), and meals on wheels service. Do accept offers of help from neighbours, friends, relatives – even if it is only to sit with the patient while you go out. You must maintain your own interests and social life if you are to be able to continue to care for more than a few weeks – if you don't look after yourself and your own needs the old demon depression may creep in!

Clubs and day centres help too

You should accept offers for your relative to attend a stroke club, day centre, or even a day ward at the local geriatric department. Despite some initial objections and excuses, patients usually benefit and may even have physio, speech, or occupational therapy sessions at these centres. Escort services to take the patient to and from day care are available in most parts of the country and are arranged by the Red Cross, the WRVS, or others (see p. 104).

Don't bottle up your feelings

It is quite common to feel frustration, anger, and resentment at the cruel blow life has struck. Some carers even feel so desperate and depressed that they resort to physical violence and strike the patient. But emotional 'violence' is more likely – particularly talking about the patient in front of him. Don't feel guilt ridden. Remember these are natural, normal reactions and don't bottle them up; discuss them with your doctor or the district nurse. Your doctor may suggest counselling, which can be very useful, or you may get help from a relatives support group, where other carers share their problems and worries (see p. 104).

Holidays should help

Carers need holidays. Arrangements can nearly always be made for a relief admission to the local authority hospital or a nursing home so that you can get a break. Some patients may 'play up' when you return, but they must learn to accept that the only way you can continue to care for them at home is by looking after your own physical and emotional health.

If you can't cope

If you become really desperate and simply cannot cope at home, your doctor will help by arranging admission to the local hospital and perhaps later, a transfer to a nursing home.

11 Risk factors for stroke

Anyone with a relative or friend who has had a stroke will wonder whether it could happen to them. A number of risk factors have been identified and there is hope that reducing these will lessen the likelihood of stroke considerably. Treating high blood pressure has been shown to be the most successful step in reducing the chance of stroke – in fact the European Working Party on High Blood Pressure in the Elderly suggests that the risk of stroke is halved. The chances of success are less certain, however, with some other treatments, for example reducing the level of cholesterol in the blood.

Factors apply to other problems

Degenerative disease of the arteries in the brain does not occur in isolation – the two other main areas where problems arise are the heart and the major arteries to the legs. The risk factors tend to be common to all three sites, but there are a few differences. For example, although there is no doubt that smoking is an important risk factor for premature heart disease, population studies have not shown convincingly that this is the case with cerebral circulation and stroke. A heart attack sometimes happens out of the blue, in someone who seems perfectly healthy.

Previous signs

Although a stroke occurs suddenly, it rarely comes unannounced and most patients have had some previous clue that there is something wrong with their arteries. Perhaps their blood pressure was high on one occasion or they have had symptoms of heart disease, like a tight pain in the chest, or symptoms of blood flow problems like pains in the calf while walking. Some people have symptoms of heart disease 10 to 15 years before their stroke.

Be aware of your body. Most stroke victims have had some previous clue of future problems.

Age

Age is by far the most important single risk factor for stroke. But don't be discouraged because this is a factor you can't change. Population studies indicate that if someone has just one risk factor working against him, this factor is not likely to increase the chances of trouble very substantially. Problems begin when the patient has two, three, or four risk factors in combination. So although we cannot change our age, we can try to rule out some of the other factors mentioned below.

High blood pressure

This is the single, most important, remediable risk factor for stroke since reducing it halves the chance of having a stroke. The number of people having strokes had started to go down, however, even before effective drugs for high blood pressure had been introduced. There have been various explanations for this, including the possibility that salt was a culprit and the population's blood pressure was falling as the salt content of the diet decreased with the introduction of refrigeration for preserving food. For the moment, it is wise to limit the amount of salt eaten. Although many people can eat a lot of salt without developing high blood pressure, others are less fortunate and more vulnerable. It is interesting to note that reducing high blood pressure has had very little effect on improving the chances of suffering heart attack.

Know your blood pressure

Although everyone should know his blood pressure, only a few of us do. Yet it is far more important for survival than knowing your height and weight. People are often confused by the two measurements given. As far as stroke prevention is concerned, the only number you need to concentrate on is the higher one (called the systolic pressure), which should ideally be 150 or less. Don't rush out and buy a blood pressure measurement machine to use yourself as this is neither necessary nor to be recommended in someone with normal blood pressure. If, however, you are being treated for high blood pressure that is difficult to control, it may be very helpful to you and your doctor to have regular, reliable measurements. Remember though to get your machine checked regularly to ensure that it is accurate!

Drug treatment

A wide variety of drugs for high blood pressure is currently available, but as some of these drugs are quite powerful it is important to introduce treatment very cautiously to avoid the possibility of dramatic falls in blood pressure when standing and after exercise.

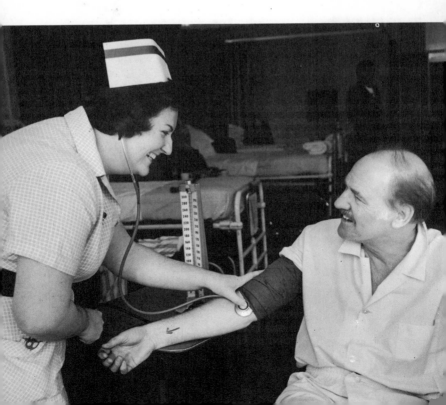

Transient cerebral ischaemic attacks

People who have suffered a transient cerebral ischaemic attack are at some risk from going on to develop a stroke. A transient ischaemic attack looks like a minor stroke as there is a disturbance of vision and speech, and weakness or loss of sensation on one side. The symptoms disappear completely within 24 hours, however, and in most cases improve within a few minutes. These attacks should be regarded as a threatened stroke and point to a risk of future circulation problems – not just strokes but also heart attacks. Someone who has had a transient ischaemic attack has approximately a 7% chance of having a serious circulatory disorder each year, untreated.

Investigation needed

It is surprising that despite the dramatic symptoms outlined, only a minority of people who have had these attacks are referred to a hospital consultant for further investigation. Very often patients are falsely reassured by the rapid recovery and are willing to accept that it was just a 'spasm' in an artery that produced the trouble, although this very rarely is the case, except in people with some kinds of migraine. Every patient who has suffered such an attack needs to be assessed and investigated fairly promptly and given the right treatment, which may be antiplatelet or anticoagulation therapy. In a few patients an operation on the major neck vessels is needed.

Heart disease

Patients with disease of the heart valves, perhaps after rheumatic fever, are prone to developing thrombi in the heart that move to the brain. This is particularly the case if the heart rhythm is abnormal. Anybody who has had palpitations or, on feeling their pulse, has noticed an irregularity which is more than just the occasional extra beat, should have this investigated.

Angina and heart failure

People with heart disease that causes a reduction in blood flow are prone to stroke. In many cases, in addition to treating their blood pressure and angina, doctors will prescribe antiplatelet therapy to prevent thrombosis and embolism. Patients with untreated heart failure are also at risk from stroke and require optimal treatment with diuretics and in some cases, enalapril or heart stimulants such as digoxin.

High cholesterol

Some people have focused on cholesterol as *the* important blood fat. But in fact it is only one of a family of fats, or lipids. Hyperlipidaemia is the name used to describe any disturbances in the way our bodies use fat and some of us have inherited a fault in handling fat. Abnormally high concentrations of cholesterol and other fats are associated with premature arterial disease and subsequent complications, like heart attack and stroke. People who have inherited this disorder may require drugs in addition to changing their diet to treat the condition and to reduce the risks of complications.

Bad diet

Most people, however, do not have an inherited defect but a bad diet. This fact has been widely publicised recently so we can be brief. In essence:

- Dairy produce needs to be limited and skimmed milk should be used instead of creamy milk. Butter, cheese, and cream should be reduced drastically.
- Fatty meats should be avoided and the amount of meat eaten reduced very substantially.
- Eggs are not as evil a food as some people think and most normal people will not do themselves any harm by eating three or four eggs per week.
- The role of sugar (except in diabetes) is often underplayed. The bodies of people who eat a lot of sweets become fat and the same is true in their blood and tissues. Refined sugar and carbohydrates should be reduced.
- Eat plenty of high fibre cereals, fruits, and vegetables.
- Eat more fish, particularly oily fish like mackerel, herring, or salmon!

Measuring fat in blood

Measuring the amount of fat in the blood is not generally of much value except in younger patients who develop problems or where there is a family history of early arterial disease. When it is performed it is necessary to take the blood test after the patient has fasted. I should emphasise that a low fat diet has not been proved to have a major effect on the development of arterial disease or stroke except in people with an inherited disturbance in fat metabolism. This may be because measures to control fat intake are taken too late – in middle age and beyond rather than in childhood, the teens and 20s.

Fat intake should be controlled in childhood, the teens and 20s.

Diabetes mellitus

Patients with diabetes are more likely to develop stroke than others and it is therefore important for the disorder to be controlled as carefully as possible. Most diabetics do not need insulin injections but can be treated by a suitable diet and drugs taken by mouth. A reduction in weight is a very good indicator of the success of the diet. Even though their urine is free of sugar if they are not losing weight or have not reached their optimal weight, the diet is not working.

Thickness of the blood

Blood has very complex and interesting properties. Normally 35 to 50% of it is cells – mainly the red blood cells which outnumber the white blood cells by 1000 to 1. Patients whose blood has more than 50% cells have a higher chance of stroke than those with normal values. The common causes of this extra thick blood are:

- Smoking. The carbon monoxide inhaled, when smoking, makes 10 to 15% of the blood cells ineffective at carrying oxygen and so the number of red cells goes up to compensate. But some patients with thick blood as a result of smoking have another complication – for reasons as yet poorly understood, they have a reduced amount of plasma.

- Diabetes. Diabetes that is poorly controlled may cause a reduction of the volume of plasma in the circulation. This has the effect of increasing red cell concentration.
- Diuretic treatment. Diuretics (water tablets) are commonly used for high blood pressure or heart failure. They reduce the plasma volume for the first week or so in everybody who takes them, but by six weeks this has returned to normal in most people. The blood may remain thicker then optimal, however, in a few and alternative treatment may be advised.

Keep a count

Everybody who is a smoker, on water tablets, or diabetic should have their concentration of blood cells measured, as should patients with symptoms of circulatory disorders. Sometimes reducing the number of cigarettes smoked or the diuretic treatment or improving diabetic control is enough to remedy the problem, but occasionally the doctor needs to resort to thinning the blood by old fashioned blood letting. When this is done, antiplatelet treatment is necessary to prevent the increased likelihood of a clot forming after blood loss (see below).

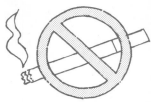

Illness or injury

When a patient is ill, for example with pneumonia or diarrhoea, or if they have just been injured, had surgery, or have lost some blood, changes occur in the blood which make it more likely to clot. This is obviously important for survival. By increasing the tendency of blood to clot, a potentially fatal blood loss occurring after injury can be prevented. It may, however, be counter-productive. To prevent unwanted thrombosis after surgery, it is quite common for antiplatelet or anticoagulant treatment to be used.

Overweight

Being slightly overweight may not be fashionable but it is probably not harmful. Those who are 20 to 30 lb overweight do not have a greatly increased chance of stroke. But people who are extremely overweight are more likely to have heart disease, high blood pressure, and stroke. Extreme overweight also makes rehabilitation after stroke much more difficult. A very heavy patient is a daunting prospect to move and to lift. A lightweight patient with a moderately weak leg may be able to get up and walk satisfactorily, whereas the heavyweight with a similar weakness may be rendered chairbound. The complications after stroke are also more likely in the overweight patient. So limiting weight is important.

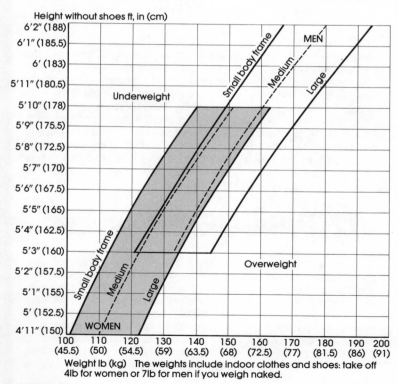

Weight chart.

Smoking

Although several population studies have failed to show that smoking is a significant risk factor for stroke, it should be emphasised that most patients studied were elderly people whose cigarette consumption was low. Perhaps the heavy smokers had been sorted out by heart disease many years before! Certainly doctors dealing with arterial disease in young and middle aged people are convinced that smoking is an important cause of this.

Why is smoking so bad?

The reasons that it is damaging are firstly, that it seems to accelerate hardening of the arteries (arteriosclerosis) and secondly, it seems to increase the likelihood of clots forming.

Do try to stop

Everyone who possibly can should stop smoking. Some people who are truly addicted to the habit, however, get so irritable, agitated and miserable, not only when coming off but when remaining off cigarettes altogether, that a compromise is required. These people may allow themselves three to five cigarettes a day, but they should make every effort to control the other risk factors. Some people attempting to stop smoking are helped by nicotine-containing chewing gum (Nicorette), which should be used whenever there is a craving for a cigarette. The chewing gum supplies the nicotine without the other harmful substances in cigarettes.

Alcohol

Alcohol is thought to have a harmful influence on the circulation of blood in the brain as well as on the brain itself. It has been shown to cause an increase in blood pressure, disturbances in the way our bodies use sugars and fats, and disturbances in blood coagulation, particularly in those who drink very heavily. These factors tend to increase the chance of stroke. Furthermore, there are considerable risks of developing thrombotic attacks particularly at the time of an alcoholic binge when the body has been considerably disrupted by loss of fluid, dehydration, and vomiting.

The oral contraceptive pill

The oral contraceptives introduced first had a high content of the hormone oestrogen, and some young women did have strokes as a result. The oestrogen content has now been reduced, however, and unless there are a number of other risk factors, taking the pill under 40 is probably safe – and certainly safer than unwanted pregnancy. Women on the pill should not smoke and the pill should be stopped if focal migraine occurs- that is migraine in which there is dysphasia, sensory problems or weakness on one side during the attack.

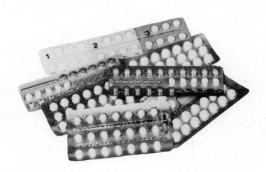

The role of stress

The role of stress in producing stroke is not very clear cut. Every doctor will have a story or two of a patient who has suffered a stroke at the time of or shortly after a period of extreme stress like bereavement, bankruptcy, or divorce.

Increased tendency to clot

The explanations for this might include an increased tendency of the blood to clot that is triggered by strains and stresses. Feelings of fear and anxiety often precede injury and activating the blood's tendency to clot would clearly reduce the blood loss.

Stress and blood pressure

Longstanding stress also causes an increase in blood pressure and is more likely to encourage other risk factors such as smoking and alcohol intake. Be reassured, however, that the human body actually copes quite well with day to day stresses and strains. When someone finds that his job has suddenly become too demanding, another explanation should be sought as there may be some underlying disturbance or problem, in many cases a mild depression.

Stress causes physical changes in the body that were useful in the past when cavemen were fleeing from dinosaurs but are often inappropriate for current day stresses like missing the train or losing your car keys down a drain.

Family history

Some people come from families where a number of members have been said to have suffered strokes and they are worried that this is going to be their inevitable fate. Firstly, strokes are common, so it is quite likely for more than one stroke to occur in families by chance. It is usually worth getting more details about the causes of death and disability in the other members of the family because you will often find that they did not have strokes after all, but heart attacks, head injuries, or tumours.

Diagnoses change

Diagnostic fashions change over the years and before modern scanning and other investigational techniques became available, patients would often be diagnosed as having stroke when this was not the case at all. Sudden death was often classified as a stroke in the past, but stroke does not cause death within seconds or minutes — even in the most severe stroke it takes some hours. Sudden death is more likely to be due to heart attacks and a disruption of heart rhythm.

Risk factors may be inherited

If it does seem that several other members of the family have suffered from a stroke, then one should ask why? The explanation is usually high blood pressure, diabetes, or a disturbance of the blood fats – factors that are inherited in some families. If this is the case measurement of blood pressure, blood sugar, and blood fats should be done. If these are normal, be strongly reassured. If abnormal, then something can be done to treat the problem and reduce the worries.

A thorough check up?

Is it necessary therefore to have a thorough check up to look into the state of the circulation in general and the circulation in the brain in particular? For most people, an expensive check up is not required. Certainly everybody should know his or her blood pressure, and urine should be checked to ensure that there is no evidence of diabetes. In those who smoke, are diabetic, or are on water pills, the concentration of the blood should be estimated. Blood fats should be checked in those who have developed symptoms of artery disease at a young age or who have a positive family history of arterial disease.

12 Preventing stroke

What can I do to prevent a stroke? This question usually arises in two situations. Firstly, in somebody who has had one and wishes to avoid another – this is called secondary prevention. Primary prevention aims to prevent a stroke in the first place. Because the appropriate advice is slightly different in the two groups I will discuss them separately.

Secondary prevention

It should be emphasised that the risk of a further stroke is not overwhelming, in fact risk of a heart attack or other medical problem is more likely. The risk is there, however, and some preventative measures are indicated. Hopefully, the question will be raised after a minor stroke when there is a lot to be gained by preventing further trouble.

One stroke does not necessarily lead to another.

Blood pressure

Again the most important risk factor to identify and treat is raised blood pressure. As mentioned earlier, this must be treated cautiously. Drugs must be introduced one at a time at a low dose and the dose gradually increased. Blood pressure treatment is not usually advised in the first two weeks after a stroke because at this time a higher pressure may be required to keep the blood flowing to the brain.

The right treatment

One needs to know whether the first stroke was a cerebral haemorrhage or an infarct. Clearly, anticoagulant drugs should not be given to a patient who has had a cerebral haemorrhage but they will benefit those who have had an infarct.

An aspirin a day . . .

Patients whose stroke was caused by thrombosis should be given aspirin as a preventive measure. Some patients may also benefit from dipyridamole, but this drug often causes headaches, particularly in migraine sufferers. The dose of aspirin required is a low one, probably 300 mg of aspirin (one standard tablet) taken three days a week will suffice. A patient with a delicate stomach can be given enteric-coated aspirin, which is less likely to produce indigestion, and if necessary aspirin suppositories.

Warfarin

Some patients with heart disorders that might lead to thrombosis can be protected by anticoagulation with warfarin. In addition, those people who continue to have transient ischaemic attacks despite aspirin should be given warfarin instead.

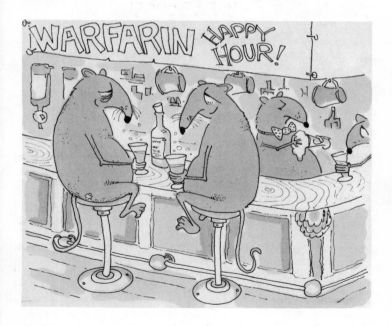

Warfarin may be bad for rats but it helps many patients.

Some problem patients

Some patients who have had peptic ulceration, intestinal bleeding, or poorly controlled blood pressure may be quite unable to take aspirin or an anticoagulant. They should be treated with dipyridamole and possibly fish oils (Maxepa). These are thought to have some action in preventing thrombosis, without provoking unnecessary bleeding.

Healthy habits

All patients should stop smoking and those who have been drinking too much alcohol should reduce their consumption to under three units a day and if they cannot achieve this, stop altogether. Those who are considerably overweight should go on a diet.

Primary prevention

Firstly, we need to consider the patient who already has a positive risk factor for stroke – he or she may have had a heart attack, a circulatory disease, high blood pressure, or diabetes. Of course, the presence of other risk factors should also be identified and treated appropriately in these patients.

Blood pressure

Most doctors agree that people under 70 with high blood pressure (over 150, systolic) should be given treatment. The evidence is good that it prevents stroke. In people over 70, however, there may be problems with side effects and the disadvantages of treatment may outweigh the possible benefits. The best policy in the elderly is to accept a slightly higher blood pressure and only to attempt treatment if the systolic blood pressure exceeds 180 in those over 70 and 200 in the over 80s. Treatment should start gently with a low dose of a diuretic and then if necessary a small dose of a calcium antagonist drug (such as nifedipine) may be added and subsequently one of a group of drugs called beta blockers (for example, atenolol). Because the arteries in some elderly people are rigid, a drop in blood pressure is accompanied by a fall in brain blood flow and they may feel lightheaded or worse as a result. If so, treatment needs to be reduced or stopped.

Blood fats

As I have already said, there is no definite evidence that the middle aged and elderly benefit from treatment unless they have a problem dealing with fat. Younger people should be advised to go on to a low saturated fat and low carbohydrate diet. Occasionally it is also necessary to take drugs (such as clofibrate, bezafibrate, and cholestyramine) to lower the harmful fats. Some preparations of fish oils (naxapa) have been shown to have an effect and most people would prefer to try this first and add one of the drugs later if necessary. Fish oils have also been shown to have an antiplatelet effect.

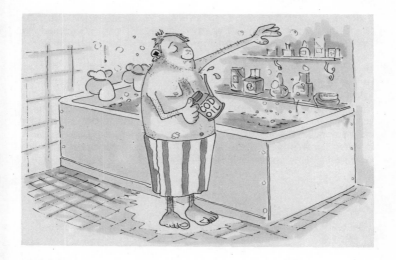

Arterial problems

Patients who have had transient cerebral ischaemic attacks or have evidence of narrowing of the carotid arteries should be investigated. In the first instance, ultrasound should be used to look at the carotid arteries. If an abnormality is found then the patient may need to have angiography (see p. 50). Patients with severe narrowing of the carotid artery may need to have surgery to treat this, but those with small amounts of narrowing can be monitored regularly. Most patients with identified risk factors should have antiplatelet treatment.

Antiplatelet treatment choices

- Aspirin: one tablet (300 mg.) per day or on alternate days using coated tablets if there is a history of indigestion.
- Fish oils: by changing diet and possibly taking Maxepa as well.
- Dipyridamole (Persantin): for those unable to tolerate aspirin.
- A combination of the above.

Change to anticoagulants

If patients continue to have transient ischaemic attacks despite antiplatelet treatment, they may need to be switched to anticoagulants such as warfarin. The dose of warfarin has to be carefully controlled so that it doubles the time taken for the blood to clot but avoids unwanted bleeding. As the dose required can vary from time to time, regular blood tests are taken (about every four to six weeks once treatment has been established). Avoid taking aspirin or any medicines containing aspirin. There is considerable interest at the moment in low dose warfarin treatment, (just 1 mg per day) as this may protect against unwanted thrombosis without any appreciable increase in the chance of bleeding.

If you are prescribed warfarin you will have regular blood tests to ensure that you are given the correct dose.

The patient with no risk factors

Some people are worried about a stroke when there are really no 'warning lights' at all. They should be reassured that although a stroke does occur suddenly, it rarely happens where there is no detectable risk factor. For their own peace of mind they should have their blood pressure checked and their blood sugar and blood fats measured. If any abnormality is found then this should be treated.

Preventive medicine

The more difficult question is whether these people would benefit from some form of treatment that prevents clots forming. For the moment, the advice should be to eat more fish and less meat and possibly to use fish oil on a regular basis. Most patients would not suffer any serious stomach problems by taking one aspirin on alternate days and I would recommend this.

Useful names and addresses

Age Concern
England – 60 Pitcairn Road, Mitcham, Surrey, CR4 3LL.
Wales – 1 Park Grove, Cardiff, CF1 3BJ.
Scotland – 33 Castle Street, Edinburgh, EH2 3DN.
Northern Ireland – 128 Great Victoria Street, Belfast, BT2 7BG.

Association of Carers, 1st Floor, 21/23 New Road, Chatham, Kent, ME4 4QJ (0634 813981).

Association of Crossroads Care Attendant Schemes Ltd. 94 Coton Road, Rugby, Warwickshire, CV21 4LN

British Red Cross, 9 Grosvenor Crescent, London, SW1X 7EJ (01 235 5454).

British School of Motoring – disabled drivers assessment units, 81-87 Hartfield Road, London, SW19 3TJ (01 540 8262).

Chest, Heart and Stroke Association, Tavistock House North, Tavistock Square, London, WC1H 9JE (01 387 3012).

Communication Aids Centre, Charing Cross Hospital, Fulham Palace Road, London W6 8RF (01 748 2040 x 3064).

Counsel and Care for the Elderly, 131 Middlesex Street, London, E1 7JF (01 621 1624).

Disabled Information Service Westminster, 10 Warwick Row, London SW1E 5EP (01 630 5994).

Disabled Living Foundation, 380–384 Harrow Road, London, W9 2HU (01 289 6111).

Help the Aged, St James's Walk, London, EC1R 1BE (01 253 0253).

Medical Adviser, D.V.L.C., Swansea, SA1 1TU.

REMAP – Engineering help for the disabled, 25 Mortimer Street, London, W1N 8AB.

Social Security Leaflets Unit, PO Box 21, Stanmore, Middlesex, HA7 1AY

- Sick or Disabled Leaflet, FB28.

Other useful leaflets*
- Leaflet NI 211 Mobility Allowance
- Leaflet NI 205 Attendance Allowance
- Leaflet H11 Fares to hospital
- Leaflet RR1 Who pays less rent and rates
- Leaflet HB1 Help for handicapped people
- Leaflet BH2 Equipment for disabled people
- Leaflet NI 244 Statutory Sick Pay – Check your rights
- Leaflet NI 16 Sickness Benefit
- Leaflet NI 16A Invalidity Benefit
- Leaflet NI 252 Severe Disablement Allowance
  * Correct at time of going to press.

SPOD (Sexual and Personal Difficulties of the Disabled), 286 Camden Road, London, N7 0BJ (01 607 8851)

Taking a break – a guide for people caring at home, Newcastle-upon-Tyne X, NE25 2AW

WRVS (Women's Royal Voluntary Service), 17 Old Park Lane, London, W1Y 4AJ (01 499 6040).

Your local Social Security Office

Glossary

Agnosia
An inability to recognise something, eg visual agnosia – an inability to recognise an object on seeing it.

Aneurysm
A swelling on an artery.

Angina
Chest, shoulder, arm pains brought on by exertion.

Apraxia
An inability to perform a task although power, coordination and sensation are preserved.

Arteriosclerosis
Hardening of the arteries.

Arteritis
An inflammation of an artery.

Arthritis
An inflammation of the joints.

Cerebral cortex
The grey matter on the surface of the brain.

Cerebral oedema
Excess water in part of the brain substance. It is usually a combination of bloated, partly damaged brain cells, bathed in extra fluid which has leaked from the circulation.

Convulsion
Usually an epileptic fit.

Digoxin
A drug from foxgloves used to treat heart failure and some irregularities of heart beat.

Diuretic
A 'water tablet' which makes you pass more urine and lowers the blood pressure.

Dysarthria
A disturbance of speech where articulation is affected. Speech is usually slurred but correct words are used and understanding is normal.

Dysphasia (aphasia) A disturbance of speech where the thought processes involved in the understanding or expression of speech are affected.

Embolism Where an artery or vein is blocked by a blood clot (usually) which has arisen elsewhere.

Embolus Usually a blood clot (but occasionally fat or air) which becomes dislodged and moves on with the circulation.

Haematoma A collection of blood that has leaked out of blood vessels.

Hemianopia Inability to see in one half of the visual field.

Hemiplegia A weakness on one side of the body.

Hyperlipidaemia Raised level of blood fats.

Hypertension High blood pressure.

Infarct Tissue damaged by interference with its blood supply.

Intermittent claudication Pains in the leg brought on by exercise, eg walking up a slope, and relieved by rest.

Lipids A group term for the blood's fats.

Myocardial infarction A heart attack.

Paraplegia A weakness of both legs.

Photophobia Irritated by light.

Pleuritic chest pain Chest pain that hurts more on taking a breath.

Seizure Any sudden attack which could include a heart attack, epilepsy or stroke.

Septicaemia Germs in the blood.

Stenosis A narrowing, in this context an artery narrowed by arteriosclerosis.

Thrombosis The process involved when blood clots.

Thrombus A blood clot.

Transient ischaemic attack

A mini-stroke that lasts less than 24 hours.

White matter

The insulated connecting fibres in the brain and spinal cord (the nervous system's wiring).

Index

age, as risk factor, 87
agnosia, 10, 36
agoraphobia, 79, 80
aids
   for driving, 83
   for hands, 70–1
   in home, 75
   mobility, 68, 69, 71
   speech, 70
alcohol, 49, 77, 94, 96, 100
aneurysm, 22, 49, 51
   Berry, 23
   and surgery, 60
anger and resentment, 43
angina, 90
angiography, 50–1, 101
anticoagulant treatment, 19, 20,
   21, 54, 55, 89, 92, 99, 102
anticonvulsants, 78
antidepressants, 42, 78
antiplatelet therapy, 19, 20, 21, 54,
   55, 78, 89, 90, 92, 102
apraxia, 10, 36
arm, 9, 30, 33, 39
arteries, 14–16, 30
   cerebral, 18
   clots in, 14, 18, 19–20
   diseased, 19
   investigation of, 49–51
   see also carotid arteries
arteriosclerosis, 14, 18, 48, 94
aspirin, 99, 102
attendance allowance, 76
attention span, short, 29, 36

balance, 13, 68, 69
bed sores, 41, 60
bladder control, 37–8, 58, 67, 77
blood
   changes in, 56
   clots, 7, 13, 14, 18, 19–20
   dilution of, 56
   disturbances, 47–8
   fats, 101
   pressure, high, 18, 24, 57, 78, 86,
      87–8, 94, 100

   pressure, low, 57
   supply, 13–16
   tests, 47–51
   thickness of, 91–2
boredom, 79
bowel control, 38, 67, 77
brain
   anatomy of, 9–16
   scan, 45–7
   stem, 9, 23, 24, 25, 28: functions
      of, 12; and surgery, 60
   tumour, 7, 17, 24
   see also cerebral
breathing difficulties, 25, 29,
   52, 61
British School of Motoring, 82

carer, support for, 42, 44, 84–5
carotid arteries, 14–16, 19, 21, 49,
   50, 101
   endarterectomy, 21, 60
catheter, urinary, 37, 58
causes, 7, 18–21, 26–7
cerebellum, 9
   functions of, 13
   and surgery, 60
cerebral
   embolism, 7, 18, 19–21, 27
   haemorrhage, 7, 22–3, 26–7, 45,
      60
   hemispheres, 9, 10–11, 23, 34,
      36, 60
   infarct, 17, 18–21, 45
   oedema, 17, 24–5, 28, 61
   thrombosis, 7, 18–19, 27
   see also brain
changes, intellectual, 79–80
Circle of Willis, 16
citizen's advice bureau, 72
clot, blood, 7, 18
   in arteries, 14, 18, 19–20
   formation of, 19
   in heart, 13, 18, 19–20
clubs for stroke sufferers, 44, 76,
   79, 84, 85
communication problems, 69–70

see also speech
computed tomogram, 45–7, 49,
    55
consciousness, 12, 13, 23, 25, 28
constipation, 77
contact, difficulty of resuming,
    80, 81
continence, 37–8, 41, 58, 67, 77
contraceptive pill, oral, 95
convulsions, 17, 42, 54, 83
coordination, 9, 13
coughing, 12, 41, 58
counselling, 42, 79, 85

death, cause of, 7, 23, 24, 25, 41
deep vein thrombosis, 41, 54
dementia, 36, 73, 82
depression, 42, 78, 84
diabetes, 18, 41, 48, 77, 91, 92
diet, 76–7, 90
disability, 10, 23, 26, 66
    see also recovery
district nurse, 76, 81, 84
diuretic therapy, 54, 92
double vision, 34
Driver and Vehicle Licensing
    Centre, 82, 83
driving, resuming, 82–3
drowsiness, 25 28, 29
dysarthria, 12, 31
dysphasia, 70, 80, 95
    jargon, 32–3

echocardiography, 51
electrocardiogram (ECG), 51
embolism
    cerebral, 7, 18, 19–21, 27
    pulmonary, 25, 41
emotional problems, 42–4, 78–9,
    83

face, 30, 31
family history as risk factor, 96–7
fat, reducing intake, 76–7, 90–1
fats in bloodstream, high, 18
fits, 17, 42, 54, 83
fluid intake, maintenance of, 53
frozen shoulder, 39, 69

general practitioner, 75–6, 78, 81

hand, use of, 30, 71
heart, 13, 18, 19–20, 54
    attack, 19, 25, 51
    disease, 89–90
    investigation of, 51
home
    assessment of, 71
    help, 76, 84
    modification to, 71, 75
    returning, 72, 73, 74–85

immobility, 25
infarct, cerebral, 17, 18–21, 26, 45
infections, 25, 58
intellectual changes, 79–80
intracerebral haemorrhage, 22

jargon dysphasia, 32–3
joints, 30, 33, 69

learned non-use, 68
leg, 9, 13, 30, 33, 54
limbs, floppy, 30

meals on wheels, 76, 84
medical social worker, 72, 73, 81
medication, 78
    see also treatment
memory problems, 29, 36
middle cerebral artery, 30
mobility aids, 68, 69, 71
morale, 43, 44, 61, 70, 73, 76, 83
movement, 10–11

nuclear magnetic resonance
    scanning, 45, 47
nursing care, 60–1, 66–7

occupational therapy, 36, 61

pain, 33–4, 39
paralysis, 12, 13, 17, 30, 31, 33, 39,
    54, 58
    one-sided, 13, 30, 31, 58
personality, altered, 43–4
physiotherapy, 36, 39, 52, 60–1,
    67–9, 72, 75
pneumonia, 25, 29, 39, 58, 69
power of attorney, 72
prevention of stroke, 98–103
    primary, 100–3

secondary, 98–100
treatment for, 49, 54, 100–3

reading difficulties, 35
recognition difficulties, 10, 35, 80
recovery, 64–73
    and nursing care, 66–7
    and occupational therapy,
        70–1, 72
    order of, 64–5
    and physiotherapy, 67–9, 72, 75
    prospects, 64
    and speech therapy, 69–70, 72,
        75
rehabilitation, 29, 61, 65, 68–73
    units, 72–3
relatives, involvement of, 68, 69
residential care, 26, 73, 74, 83
risk factors for stroke, 86–93

self-help groups, 44, 76, 79, 84, 85
sensory disturbances, 11, 12, 33–4,
    95
series of strokes, 36, 45, 52
sex after stroke, 83
sight problems, 10–11, 26, 34–6
    and brain stem, 12
    loss of vision, 36
site of stroke, 23, 30, 45–7
size of stroke, 23, 45–7
smoking, 91–2, 94, 95, 96
spasm, 23
spasticity, 30, 68
speech, 10–11, 12
    aids, 70
    disturbance, 21, 26, 31–3, 81
    therapy, 31, 61, 69–70, 72, 75
spinal cord, 9
state benefits, 72
steroid treatment, 24, 39
stress, as risk factor, 19, 95–6
subarachnoid haemorrhage, 22,
    47, 49
support after returning home,
    74–6
support for carer, 42, 44, 84–5
surgery, 14, 19, 21, 22, 49, 58–60,
    89, 101
swallowing, 12, 23, 29, 39, 61
    treatment for, 52

symptoms, 21, 22, 26–7, 86, 89

talking see speech
therapy, specialist, 60–1
    see also under individual
        names
thought processes, damaged,
    31–3, 80
thrombosis, 7, 18–19, 27
    deep vein, 41, 54
    and surgery, 60
toileting, regular, 38, 58
transient ischaemic attack, 21, 26,
    55, 82, 89, 99, 101, 102
treatment, 45, 52–63
    aims of, 52
    for blood pressure, 88
    for formation of clots, 19
    future, 62–3
    for high cholesterol and fats,
        90–1
    preventive, 49, 54, 100–3
    surgical, 14, 19, 21, 22
trembling, 13

ultrasound techniques, 49, 51
unconsciousness, 28
understanding, 10–11
    difficulty with, 31–2
    of problems, 42
urinary infection, 25, 58
use of affected parts, 67–8, 71
    see also paralysis
    physiotherapy

vertebral arteries, 14–16, 49, 50
violence, 84–5
voluntary organisations, 84, 104

walking, 13, 30, 68, 69
warfarin, 99
weakness, 21, 26, 29–30, 95
    patterns of, 30
weight
    chart, 8, 93
    problems, 76–7
    as risk factor, 93
work, return to, 81